THE OFFICIAL
U.S. ARMY
POCKET
PHYSICAL
TRAINING
GUIDE

GET **ARMY FIT**: BUILD **STRENGTH**, **MOBILITY**, **ENDURANCE** & **HEALTH**

United States Army

The Official US Army Pocket Physical Training Guide

Get Army Fit: Build Strength, Mobility, Endurance and Health

U.S. Army

This edition first published 2017 by Carlile Military Library. "Carlile Military Library" and its associated logos and devices are trademarks. Carlile Military Library is an imprint of Carlile Media. The appearance of U.S. Department of Defense (DoD) visual information does not imply or constitute DoD endorsement.

Published in the United States of America.

ISBN-13: 978-1-9794-0198-2
ISBN-10: 1979401985

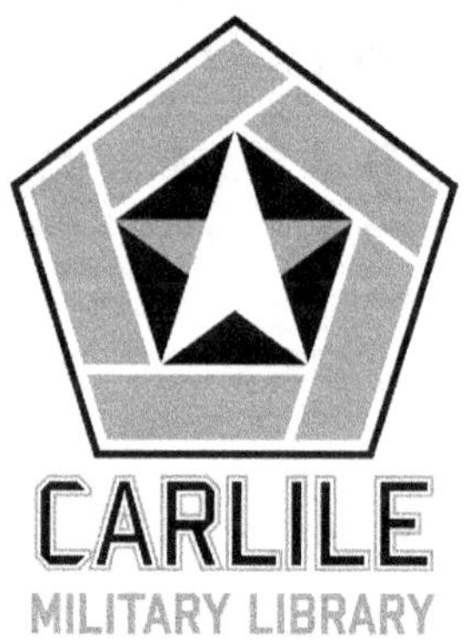

Pocket Physical Training Guide

This publication contains the following information:

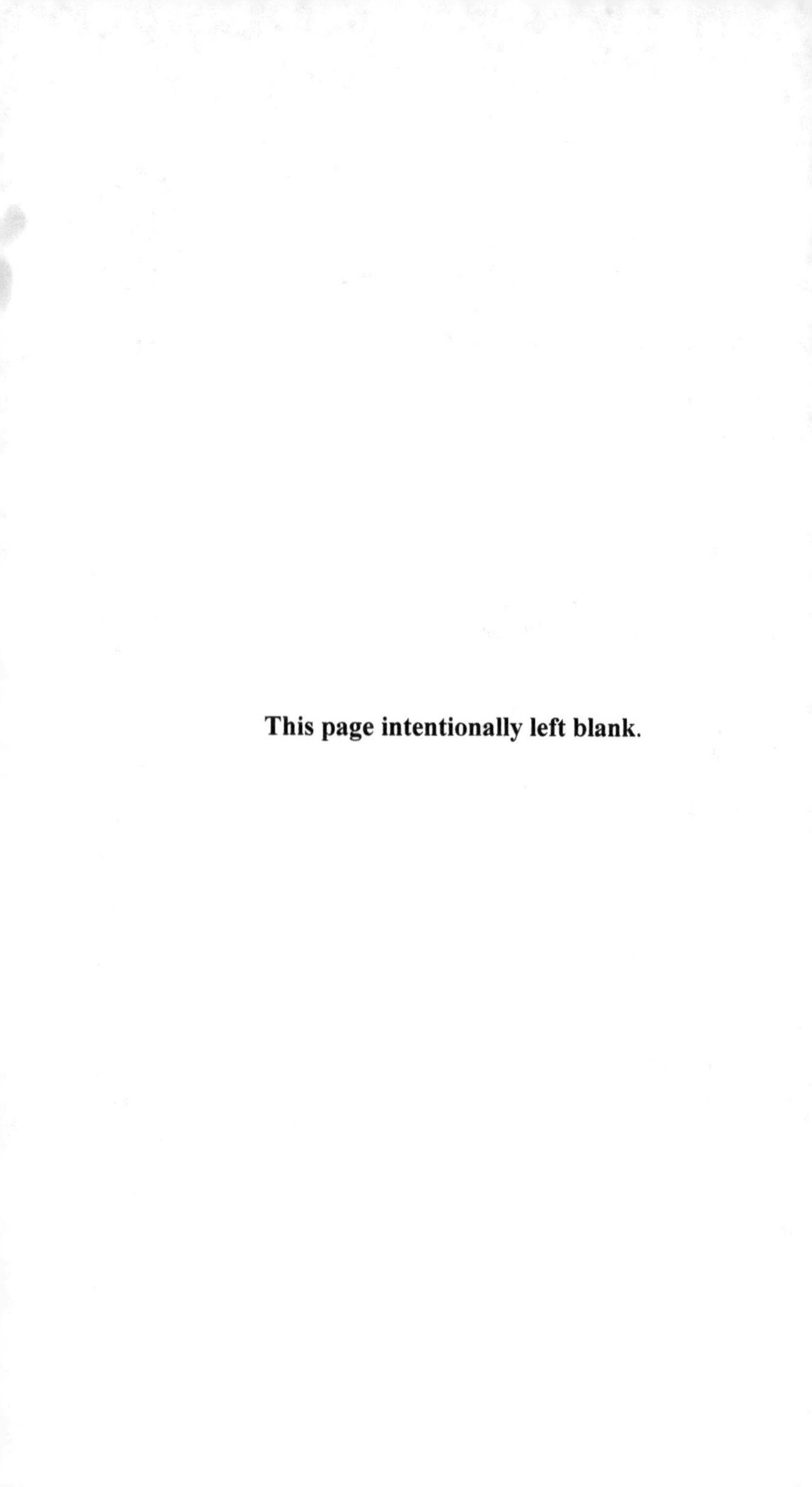

This page intentionally left blank.

INTRODUCTION

The following information is provided for individuals preparing for the physical demands of Initial Military Training (IMT). The staff of the U.S. Army Physical Fitness School (USAPFS) prepared this Pocket Physical Training Guide. This document is the sole property of United States Army Training and Doctrine Command (TRADOC) and is intended for use by U.S. Army Recruiters to assist future Soldiers.

This guide was written in recognition that both the quality and quantity of physical activity recommended to the individuals using this guide is consistent with current physical activity recommendations for the general public. The fitness components of Cardiorespiratory endurance, muscular strength and endurance, flexibility, and body composition are all inherent within this generalized exercise prescription. This program specifies the intensity, duration, and frequency of training, and it is the interaction of these three variables that results in improved health and physical fitness.

In order for this program to be safe and effective, it must be followed as written. Exercise must be conducted regularly at the proper intensity to bring about the desired changes in the body. However, changes in the body occur gradually; so be patient and adhere to the program. If you miss a session for some reason, just pick up where you left off with the next day's session. However, if you miss a whole week of sessions, you will have to start the week over. In addition, following the nutritional guidance in this document and ensuring adequate rest and recovery will optimize health, improve physical fitness, and control injuries.

DO NOT begin this physical exercise program before passing a routine physical examination at the Military Entrance Processing Station (MEPS).

GETTING STARTED

Your physical training program will begin with an assessment of
your present physical condition. Your Recruiter will administer an
assessment (the 1-1-1 Physical Fitness Assessment), which consists of
one minute of push-ups, one minute of sit-ups, and a timed, one-mile
run. This assessment will determine your starting point and appropriate
placement in the Pre-BCT Standardized Physical Training Program. You
and your Recruiter will review your scores to determine which training
schedule you will follow. Commit to spending approximately 45 minutes
per day, four to five times a week in the conduct of physical training.
Whether you follow the walk-to-run guidelines or begin training at
a higher level, this program will help prepare you for the physical
requirements of IMT. If you follow this training program, you will
experience many of the health-related benefits of physical activity.

Adherence to the Pre-BCT Physical Training Program begins your
preparation for the successful completion of the IMT graduation
requirement to pass the Army Physical Fitness Test (APFT). This test
consists of two minutes of push-ups, two minutes of sit-ups, and a
timed, two-mile run. Performance standards are based on age and
gender.

Safety Considerations

The Pre-BCT Program is a safe and effective way to improve your
physical fitness. To achieve these results, it must be followed as written.

- ALWAYS perform the prescribed warm-up and cool-down before and
  after the training activity.
- Perform ONLY the prescribed number of sets and repetitions on the
  training schedule.

- Proper form (precision) is more important than the sloppy execution of more repetitions.
- Perform ALL the exercises in the order listed for each drill.
- If you miss a day of training, pick up with the next day of the training schedule.
- Exercise with a training partner whenever possible.

Although a little muscle soreness is to be expected when beginning a new physical training program, do not aggravate injuries by continuing to exercise when you are feeling pain or discomfort.

Injury Control

Injuries are not uncommon during intense physical training. Most injuries can, however, be prevented. Safety is always a major concern.

Many common injuries are caused by overuse, that is, exercising too much and too often and with too rapid an increase in the workload. Most overuse injuries can be treated with rest, ice, compression and elevation.

The most common running injuries occur in the feet, ankles, knees and legs. Although they are hard to eliminate, much can be done to keep them to a minimum. Preventive measures include proper warm-up and cool-down. Failure to allow recovery between hard bouts of running can lead to overtraining and can also be a major cause of injuries. If you experience continuing or acute pain, see your doctor.

Shoes

Proper footwear may play a role in injury prevention. Choosing a running shoe that is suitable for your particular type of foot can help you avoid some common running-related injuries. It can also make running more enjoyable and help you get more mileage out of your shoes.

- Always tie and untie shoes when putting them on and taking them off.
- Expect shoes to be comfortable when you try them on. If they are not, then do not buy them.
- How a shoe looks is not as important as proper fit or comfort.
- Replace running shoes when they begin to show visible wear or after 500 miles of use, whichever occurs first.
- The best shoe for you may not be the most expensive. Always try on both shoes and walk around the store to ensure they fit before purchasing.
- If possible, shop for shoes at the end of the day instead of in the morning. Your feet swell from being in shoes and moving around all day.

Clothing

Proper clothing can also help prevent injuries.

- Ensure that you are wearing some sort of reflective material if exercising during hours of low visibility.

- Clothes should be comfortable, light in color, and fit loosely in warm weather.

- Clothing may be layered according to personal preference in cold weather and gloves or mittens and ear-protecting caps should be worn to prevent frostbite.

- Rubberized or plastic suits should NEVER be worn during exercise or the physical assessments.

Environmental Conditions

- Do not exercise in extremely hot or cold weather; try to find an alternate indoor location to reduce the risk of heat or cold injuries.

- Avoid exercising near heavily traveled streets and highways during peak traffic hours.

- Avoid exposure to pollutants before and during exercise, if possible (including tobacco).

- In areas of high smog concentrations, train early in the day or later in the evening.

- Use a waterproof or sweat proof sunblock when exercising in warm weather to avoid sunburn. Follow the instructions on the bottle for proper use.

Signs and Symptoms of Heat Injuries

If you experience any of the below symptoms of heat cramps, heat exhaustion, or heatstroke, immediately stop your physical activity.

Heat Cramps
Muscular Twitching
Cramping
Muscular Spasms in Arms, Legs or Abdomen

Heat Exhaustion (Requires Medical Attention)
Excessive Thirst
Fatigue
Lack of Coordination
Increased Sweating
Cool/Wet Skin
Dizziness and/or Confusion

Heatstroke (MEDICAL EMERGENCY, DIAL 911)
No Sweating
Hot/Dry Skin
Rapid Pulse
Rapid Breathing
Coma
Seizure
Dizziness and/or Confusion
Loss of Consciousness

Signs and Symptoms of Cold Weather Injuries

During exercise in the cold, your body usually produces enough heat to maintain its normal temperature. As you get fatigued, however, you slow down and your body produces less heat. Hypothermia develops when the body cannot produce heat as fast as it is losing it.

Hypothermia
Shivering
Loss of Judgment
Slurred Speech
Drowsiness
Muscle Weakness

Frostbite
A white or grayish-yellow skin area

Skin that feels unusually firm or waxy

Numbness in body parts exposed to the cold such as the nose, ears, feet, hands, and skin

Hydration

Water is the preferred hydration fluid before, during and after physical training activities in the Pre-BCT program.

- Drink 13 to 20 ounces of cool water at least 30-60 minutes before beginning exercise (approximately 2 glasses of water).

- After the activity, drink to satisfy thirst, then drink a little more.

- After exercise, avoid alcoholic beverages and soft drinks because they are not suitable for proper hydration and recovery. Sports drinks may be consumed, but are not required and contain a considerable number of additional calories.

- It is also possible to drink too much water. Be sure to limit intake to NO MORE THAN 1 1/2 quarts per hour (48 oz.) during heavy exertion.

Nutrition

In addition to exercise, proper nutrition plays a major role in attaining and maintaining total fitness. Good dietary habits greatly enhance your ability to perform at your maximum potential. A good diet alone, however, will not make up for poor health and exercise habits.

Your body needs carbohydrates, protein, some fat, vitamins, minerals, fiber, and water to be healthy and grow strong. Include foods from each of the main food groups in your diet to get all the nutrients you need.

Bread, Cereal, Rice, and Pasta

What do you get? Carbohydrate, vitamins, minerals, fiber, and a small amount of protein.

Try to make at least half of your choices whole-grain products, such as 100 percent whole grain bread, brown rice or wild rice, barley, or oatmeal.

Vegetables

What do you get? Carbohydrate, vitamins, minerals, fiber, and a small amount of protein.

Eat lots of different ones – at least 3 to 5 servings a day, especially deep green types and the red, yellow, and orange varieties.

Fruit

What do you get? Carbohydrate, vitamins, minerals, and fiber.

Eat all varieties – at least 2 a day. Try to have a citrus fruit or juice (for example orange or grapefruit) plus a blue, red, purple, or orange type (such as blueberries, strawberries, plums or peaches) every day.

Milk, Yogurt, and Cheese

What do you get? Protein, carbohydrate in milk and yogurt, vitamins, and minerals (especially calcium).

Select 1 percent or nonfat milk or cottage cheese, nonfat or low-fat yogurt and part-skim or fat-reduced cheeses.

Meats, Poultry, Fish, Eggs, Nuts, Dry Beans

What do you get? Protein, vitamins and minerals (especially iron and zinc) plus carbohydrate in beans.

Choose lean meats (ones with the words "round," "loin," or "leg" in the name), skinless chicken or turkey breast, ham, any fish or seafood (if not fried or in butter), egg whites, and veggie burgers.

Fats, Oils, and Sweets

What do you get? Mostly extra calories.

A little is all right, but it's easy to get too much. Cut way back on fried, greasy, oily, creamy, and buttery foods. Limit high-sugar, nutrient poor foods like candy, desserts, and sugar-sweetened soda pop and fruit drinks to once in a while and in small amounts.

Nutrition Tips

- ❏ At least two-thirds of your plate should be covered with foods from the grains, vegetables, and fruits groups and no more than one third should have a low-fat or lean protein source from the milk or meat group.

- ❏ To lose weight, decrease calories while increasing exercise and activity. You can decrease calories by decreasing portions and limiting high-fat and high-sugar and nutrition-poor foods.

- ❏ To gain weight, slightly increase calorie consumption while starting your resistance training program to gain muscle not fat.

- ❏ Avoid most fast foods and processed foods (such as burgers and sausage, chips, fries and other deep-fried foods, snack crackers, snack cakes, and pastries).

- ❏ Drink 8-10 glasses of water a day.

- ❏ Take a "food first" approach to achieving good health and performance. If you feel you are unable to meet your nutritional needs through your diet, consider taking a daily multi-vitamin, multi-mineral supplement that contains no more than 100 percent of the Recommended Daily Allowance.

If you have questions, consult a registered nutritionist or dietitian.

STANDARDIZED PHYSICAL TRAINING SESSION

A standardized physical training session consists of three essential elements: warm-up, activity, and cool-down. These elements are integrated to produce the desired training effect. More importantly, every standardized physical training session must have a specific purpose. This purpose, to prepare you for the physical demands of IMT, follows a recommended rate of progression, specific to each individual's tolerance to the current level of training. There are three stages of standardized progression: initial, improvement, and maintenance.

The initial conditioning stage includes light muscular endurance activities and moderate-level Cardiorespiratory endurance activities that produce minimal muscle soreness and control injuries. This stage usually lasts up to four weeks and is dependent upon the individual's adaptation to exercise. The duration of the main activity during the initial stage will begin with approximately 15 to 20 minutes and may progress to 30 minutes. Individual goals are established by your Recruiter early in your exercise program and are reflected in where you start in the training schedule. These goals are realistic and provide personal rewards. The initial stage is the Walk-to-Run Program and the muscular strength and endurance sessions conducted in weeks one through four.

The goal of the improvement stage is to provide a gradual increase in the overall exercise stimulus to allow for more significant improvements in your fitness level. As an example, you will exercise at a moderate to vigorous intensity for 20 to 30 minutes continuously. This is shown through the increased running times in the running progression and the increased number of sets and repetitions in Conditioning Drill 2 and Conditioning Drill 3.

The goal of the maintenance stage is the long-term maintenance of the Cardiorespiratory and muscular strength and endurance fitness developed during the weeks spent in the improvement stage. This stage of the standardized physical fitness training program begins when you have reached the pre-established fitness goals set by your Recruiter.

Your exercise program will incorporate levels of intensity, frequency, and duration consistent with the objective of preparing you physically for the challenges of IMT. All standardized physical training sessions in this program have been developed using this model. Your Recruiter will guide you through the 12-week PRE-BCT Standardized Physical Training Schedule, and he or she will monitor your performance with periodic assessments. Your Recruiter will provide instruction to you regarding your participation in this program. As an example, your Recruiter will assess your fitness level with the 1-1-1 Physical Fitness Assessment.

Warm-up Exercise Drills
The standardized physical training session will always include the following elements: warm-up, activity and cool-down. The warm-up should last approximately 15 minutes and occur just before the activities of the physical training session. On training days that concentrate primarily on strength and mobility, the performance of 4 for the Core and the Hip Stability Drill should be conducted, followed by Conditioning Drill 1. On training days that concentrate primarily on endurance and mobility, the warm-up consists of the performance of Conditioning Drill 1, followed by The Military Movement Drill. After the warm-up, you are prepared for more vigorous conditioning activities. Optimal musculoskeletal function requires that an adequate range of motion be maintained at all joints. The dynamic exercises contained in each of the warm-up drills challenge the body's range of motion to achieve a variety of postures.

4 for the Core	
1. The Bent-leg Raise	(hold for 60 seconds)
2. The Side Bridge	(hold for 60 seconds)
3. The Back Bridge	(hold for 60 seconds)
4. The Quadraplex	(hold for 60 seconds)

See 4 for the Core tab.

The Hip Stability Drill	
1. The Lateral Leg Raise	(5 repetitions on each side)
2. The Medial Leg Raise	(5 repetitions on each side)
3. The Lateral Bent-leg Raise	(5 repetitions on each side)
4. The Single-leg Tuck	(5 repetitions on each side)
5. The Single-leg Over	(hold for 20 seconds on each side)

See Hip Stability Drill tab.

Conditioning Drill 1

Conditioning Drill 1	
1. The Bend and Reach	(5 repetitions - slow)
2. The Rear Lunge	(5 repetitions - slow)
3. The High Jumper	(5 repetitions - moderate)
4. The Rower	(5 repetitions - slow)
5. The Squat Bender	(5 repetitions - slow)
6. The Windmill	(5 repetitions - slow)
7. The Forward Lunge	(5 repetitions - slow)
8. The Prone Row	(5 repetitions - slow)
9. The Bent-leg Body Twist	(5 repetitions - slow)
10. The Push-up	(5 repetitions - moderate)

See Conditioning Drill 1 tab.

The Military Movement Drill

The Military Movement Drill	
1. Verticals	(1 repetition)
2. Laterals	(1 repetition)
3. The Shuttle Sprint	(1 repetition)

See Military Movement Drill tab.

Standardized Physical Training Activities

The activities of your standardized physical training session (speed running, sustained running, Conditioning Drill 2, and Conditioning Drill 3) are specified on the physical training schedule. See training schedules tab for speed running, sustained running, Conditioning Drill 2 and Conditioning Drill 3 tabs.

Standardized Cool-down

The cool-down serves to gradually slow the heart rate and helps prevent pooling of the blood in the legs and feet. You should begin the cool-down by walking until your heart rate returns to less than 100 beats per minute (BPM) and heavy sweating stops.

The cool-down should last approximately 10 minutes and occur immediately after the activities of the standardized physical training session. The performance of The Stretch Drill makes up the cool-down for ALL physical training sessions. The cool-down safely brings you back to your pre-exercise state after performing vigorous conditioning activities. The Stretch Drill provides exercises that are designed to improve flexibility in most major muscle groups of the body. These static stretches involve slowly stretching muscles and then holding that position for an extended period of time.

The Stretch Drill	
1. The Overhead Arm Pull	(hold for 20 seconds on each side)
2. The Rear Lunge	(hold for 20 seconds on each side)
3. The Extend and Flex	(hold for 20 seconds in each stretch position)
4. The Thigh Stretch	(hold for 20 seconds on each side)
5. The Single-leg Over	(hold for 20 seconds on each side)

See Stretch Drill tab.

RUNNING
(Cardiorespiratory Endurance Training)

Cardiorespiratory endurance refers to your body's ability to utilize oxygen in the working muscles. IMT will challenge your Cardiorespiratory endurance in activities such as: ability group runs, speed running, foot marching, obstacle and bayonet assault course negotiation, and common skills training.

GETTING STARTED

You and your Recruiter will review the results of the one-mile run event on the 1-1-1 Physical Fitness Assessment. Your one-mile run time will be used to determine your placement in either the Walk-to-Run Program or one of the three running ability groups (A, B or C). Your Recruiter will inform you of which training schedule to follow and the running ability group to which you will be assigned. See Training Schedules tab. When beginning a running program, care should be taken to follow a proper progression for both intensity and duration. Cardiorespiratory training, particularly running, if begun without proper preparation can contribute to lower extremity injuries. Improvements in your body's ability to use oxygen occur when exercise involves the use of large muscle groups over extended periods in activities that are rhythmic and aerobic in nature (e.g., running, walking, swimming, cycling, and some recreational sports). Walking or running may be the activity of choice because it is readily accessible and can be performed any time or place with little or no training.

Walk-to-Run Program

If you are a male and your one-mile time was slower than 8:30 or
a female and your one-mile time was slower than 10:30 on the 1-1-1
Physical Fitness Assessment, begin with this section. When new runners
or runners of lower fitness levels start a running program, they often
follow a walk-run progression. During the first four weeks, you will
alternate walking and running for the time listed on the training
schedule and repeat the walk-run routine five times in each training
session. You will gradually decrease the walk time and increase the run
times over the four weeks. When you have completed the walk-to-run
program, you are ready to progress to the next stage of your training.
The run progression starts at week 5 of your designated training
schedule. You should run continuously for the time period listed on the
training schedule. You should run at a pace that you are able to maintain
for the entire time listed. You should not feel out of breath during the
runs. If you are able to carry on a conversation as you run (the talk test),
then you are probably running at the right pace. Resist the temptation
to run longer than the time period listed on the training schedule. The
program will get harder; it is designed to gradually and safely increase
your endurance. During weeks seven through 12, you will run one mile
at a designated pace that progresses each week to enable you to meet
the BCT standard. You will also add speed running to the program, which
will increase the intensity and help you to run faster. Make sure that you
properly warm up with the standardized warm-up before the walk-run
activity. Refer to the training schedules at Training Schedules tab.

Sustained Running

If you are a male and your one-mile time was 8:30 or faster or a female
and your one-mile time was 10:30 or faster on the 1-1-1 Physical Fitness
Assessment, begin with this section. Run continuously for the time
period, at the designated pace listed for your gender and ability group,
on the training schedule. The program will get harder; it is designed

to gradually and safely increase your endurance. You will also add speed running to the program, which will increase the intensity and help you to run faster with improved running form. Make sure that you properly warm up with the standardized warm-up before running and properly cool down with the standardized cool-down after the running activity. The following table displays running ability groups categorized by one-mile run times and gender. For example, if a female ran the one-mile run event in 9:30, she would be placed in Female Ability Group B. Refer to the training schedules at Training Schedules tab.

Sustained Running Ability Groups			
GENDER	A	B	C
MALE	7:00 or faster	7:01 - 7:45	7:46 - 8:30
FEMALE	8:31 - 9:00	9:01 - 9:45	9:46 - 10:30

NOTE: If a female runs faster than the female run times listed above, the Recruiter will select the appropriate male running ability group, and she will run at the male pace times listed on the training schedules at Training Schedules tab.

Speed Running

Speed running will help you to improve your fitness level in a relatively short time and increase your running speed. In speed running, you will alternate periods of fast running with periods of walking. In this way, you can do more fast-paced running in a given workout than if you continuously run without resting. During speed running, you will perform a work interval (run fast) in a specified time for a specific number of repetitions. The work intervals are followed immediately by an active recovery interval (walk). Speed running improves the active muscles' resistance to fatigue by repeatedly exposing them to high intensity effort. An appropriate work to recovery ratio for improving speed is 1:2. You will perform speed work in the form of 30:60s, adhering to a work to recovery ratio of 1:2. During the work (run) interval, you will sprint for 30 seconds. During the recovery (walk) interval, you will walk for 60 seconds. This is one repetition of 30:60s. Speed running is performed once a week, starting week one, continuing to the end of the 12-week program. You will progress from four to 10 repetitions of speed running intervals.

Running Form

Running form varies from person to person. Differences in body types, i.e., limb lengths and muscle balance, may cause individuals to have variations in their running style. Attempts to force an individual to conform to one standard may do more harm than good. However, there are some basic guidelines that may improve running efficiency without overhauling the individual's natural stride. Generally, the form and technique for all types of running are fairly constant. The following information addresses optimal running form for the major body segments.

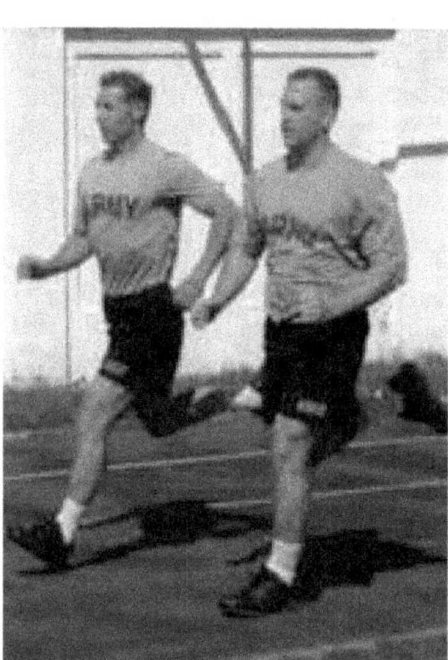

Refer to the figure at left.

Head

The head should be held high, with the chin neither pointing up nor down. Allowing the head to ride forward puts undue strain on the muscles of the upper back.

Shoulders

The shoulders should assume a neutral posture, neither rounded forward nor forcefully arched backward. Rounding the shoulders forward is the most common fault in everyday posture as well as with running. This is usually associated with tightness of the chest and shoulder muscles. Another problem occurs when the shoulders start to rise with fatigue or increased effort. This position not only wastes energy, but can also adversely affect breathing.

Arms

Throughout the arm swing, the elbows should stay at roughly a 90-degree bend. The wrists stay straight and the hands remain loosely cupped with palms facing inward. The arm swing should be free of tension, but do not allow the hands to cross the midline of the body.

Trunk and Pelvis

The trunk should remain over its base of support, the pelvis. A common problem with fatigue is allowing the trunk to lean forward of the legs and pelvis. This forces the lower back muscles to spend too much energy resisting further trunk collapse to the front.

Legs

For sustained running, much of the power is generated from below the knee. Energy is wasted as the knees come higher and the large muscles around the hips and thighs are engaged. While running, concentrate on getting a strong push-off from the ankle of the back leg. This helps to naturally lengthen the stride. Lengthening the stride by reaching forward with the front leg will be counterproductive.

Feet

The feet should be pointing directly forward while running. With fatigue and certain muscle imbalances, the legs and feet will start to rotate outward. This may hinder performance and create abnormal stresses that contribute to injury.

Breathing

Breathing should be rhythmic in nature and coordinated with the running stride.

CALISTHENICS
(Strength and Mobility Training)

Strength runs a continuum between muscular strength and muscular endurance. Muscular Strength refers to your ability to overcome maximum resistance in one single effort. Muscular Endurance refers to the ability to overcome sub-maximal resistance in repeated efforts over a period of time. Mobility is the functional application of strength and endurance. IMT will challenge your strength, mobility and endurance on obstacle courses, buddy carries, the bayonet assault course, foot marches, and during daily activities that involve lifting. Criteria for placement of Soldiers in Training Schedules 3 and 4 (push-up and/or sit-up failure) is listed below.

Males: less than 13 push-ups and/or less than 17 sit-ups
Females: less than 3 push-ups and/or less than 17 sit-ups

GETTING STARTED

Strength and Mobility Training does not require a gym or expensive equipment. In fact, it is best to start with just the resistance of your own body to develop proper form. Calisthenic exercises can be performed at home in a relatively small space and in a time-efficient manner. Calisthenics are an integral part of this fitness program for muscular strength and mobility. In addition to the development and maintenance of muscular strength, the physiological benefits of resistance training include increases in bone mass and in the strength of connective tissue. This is particularly important to establish injury control in the beginning stages of an exercise program. The conditioning drills that you will follow in this program consist of exercises that train the major muscle groups of the arms, shoulders, chest, abdomen, back, hips, and legs.

The primary goal of this training is to develop total body strength and mobility in a relatively time-efficient manner. These calisthenic exercises should be performed on alternate days; additional sets and repetitions will bring about larger strength gains.

Conditioning Drill 1

Conditioning Drill 1 (CD1) consists of a variety of calisthenics that develop motor skills while challenging strength, endurance, and flexibility. The exercises in the drill are always performed in the sequence listed below. Conditioning Drill 1 is always used in the conduct of the warm-up.

Conditioning Drill 1

1. The Bend and Reach
2. The Rear Lunge
3. The High Jumper
4. The Rower
5. The Squat Bender
6. The Windmill
7. The Forward Lunge
8. The Prone Row
9. The Bent-leg Body Twist
10. The Push-up

For a complete explanation, see Conditioning Drill 1 tab.

Conditioning Drill 2

Conditioning Drill 2 (CD2) is designed to enhance upper body strength, endurance, and mobility. As in Conditioning Drill 1, all exercises are to be performed in the sequence listed. You should try to find a partner(s) to assist you, when performing the Pull-ups. Conditioning Drill 2 consists of the following exercises:

> **Conditioning Drill 2**
>
> 1. The Push-up
> 2. The Sit-up
> 3. The Pull-up

For a complete explanation, see Conditioning Drill 2 tab. For more information on the hand position for the Pull-up, see below.

Hand Position

The overhand grip is the grip used for the pull-up. The hands are placed shoulder width apart with thumbs around the bar for the overhand grip.

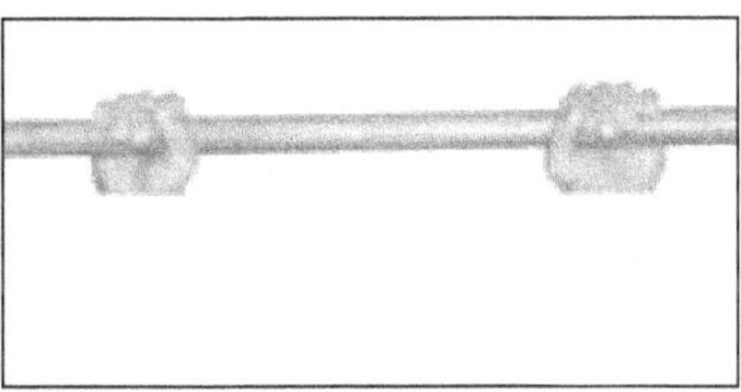

Overhand Grip

Conditioning Drill 3

Conditioning Drill 3 (CD3) consists of five higher-level toughening phase exercises that develop more complex motor skills while challenging strength, endurance, and mobility at a higher intensity. All of the exercises in the drill are conducted to cadence, and are always performed in the sequence listed. Exercises are performed to cadence for five 4-count repetitions, progressing to 10 repetitions. Precise execution should never be sacrificed for speed.

> **Conditioning Drill 3**
>
> 1. The Power Jump
> 2. The V-up
> 3. The Mountain Climber
> 4. The Leg Tuck and Twist
> 5. The Single-leg Push-up

For a complete explanation, see Conditioning Drill 3 tab.

<h1 style="text-align:center">Stability Training</h1>

Stability is dependent on structural strength and body management. Regular precise performance of 4 for the Core and The Hip Stability Drill form a foundation of good stability for physical performance. The exercises in these drills may be performed prior to Conditioning Drill 1 during the warm-up and/or after cool-down. These drills may also be performed separate from the regular training sessions as supplemental training. DO NOT exceed 60 seconds for each 4 for the Core exercise and perform NO MORE THAN 10 repetitions of Exercises 1 through 4 of The Hip Stability Drill. DO NOT EXCEED 60 seconds for Exercise 5 of The Hip Stability Drill. If performance of more repetitions is desired, don't single out any one exercise to be repeated. Instead, repeat each or both of these drills in their entirety.

4 FOR THE CORE

The abdomen, lower spine and pelvis comprise the trunk (core) of the body. This area must be stable so the limbs have a fixed base from which to create powerful movements. The abdominal and back muscles form a supportive ring around the spine. You are only as strong as your weakest link. So we must train all these muscles in a manner that mimics their function. The commands for 4 for the Core are: "Starting Position, MOVE", "Ready, EXERCISE." 4 for the Core exercises follow.

THE BENT-LEG RAISE

Lying in the Starting Position for the sit-up, place the fingers of both hands underneath the small of the back. Raise the feet off of the ground until both the hips and knees are flexed to 90 degrees. Next, contract the abdominals as if you are preparing for a blow to the stomach. Another way to perform this drawing-in maneuver is to imagine pulling the navel toward the spine. Think about the amount of pressure on your fingers created by the contraction of your abdominals. Maintain the same degree of pressure as you slowly straighten the legs. As soon as you can no longer maintain the same degree of pressure on your fingers, bring the legs back to the Starting Position and repeat until one minute has elapsed.

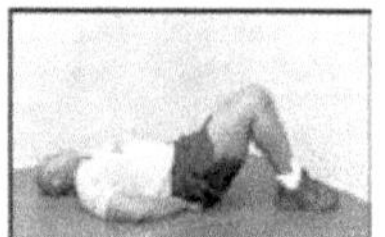

Starting
Position

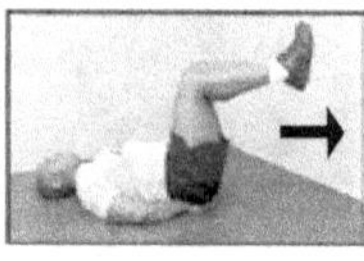

The Bent-leg Raise

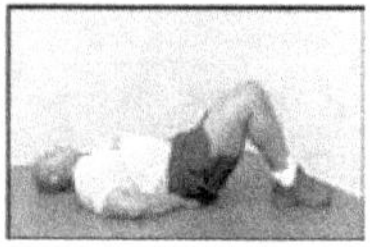

Starting
Position

THE SIDE BRIDGE

Lay on your side with your upper body off the ground, supported by
the upper body with the elbow, forearm, and fist. Cross the bottom
leg in front of the top leg, with the feet together. The legs may also be
positioned with the knees together and knees bent 90 degrees. Firmly
press into the ground with the supporting arm, then raise the trunk
and pelvis straight upward until they form a straight line with the
legs/knees. Hold this position while continuing to breathe. Switch to
the other side after one minute. If you cannot hold for one minute,
lower, rest briefly, then repeat until one minute has elapsed.

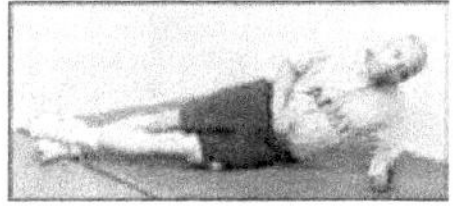

Starting Position (Left)

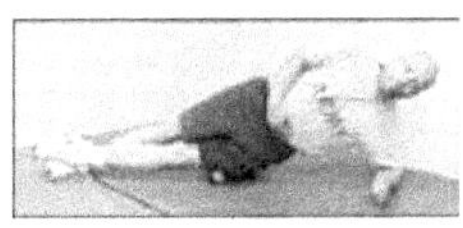

Left Side Bridge

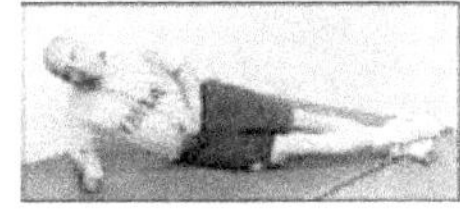

Starting Position (Right)

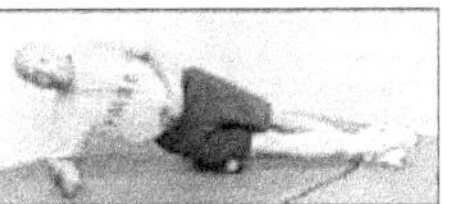

Right Side Bridge

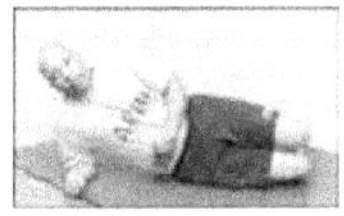

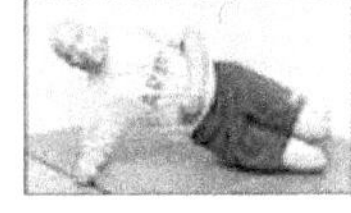

Modified Side Bridge (on knees)

THE BACK BRIDGE

Lying on the back with knees bent to 90 degrees, arms extended sideward at 45 degrees and feet on the marching surface, perform the drawing-in maneuver. Once the abdominal contraction is established, raise the hips off of the ground until the trunk and thighs form a generally straight line. The spine must not arch to achieve this position. With the buttocks still up, straighten the left leg until it comes in line with the trunk and thigh. Don't let the trunk and pelvis sag on the unsupported side. Hold five seconds, then switch to the other leg. Repeat for one minute. If the spine begins to sag, arch, or tilt, lower to the Starting Position, rest for 3-5 seconds, then, try again.

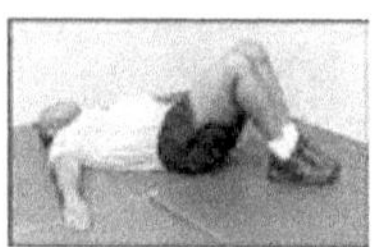

Starting Position

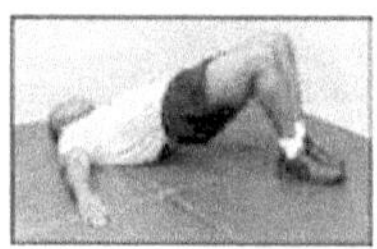

Back Bridge Position

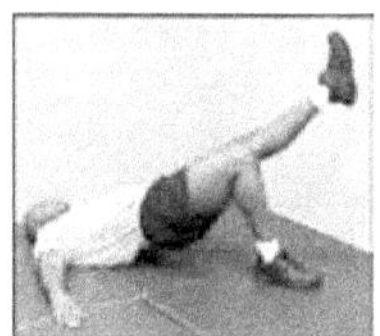

Left Leg Back Bridge

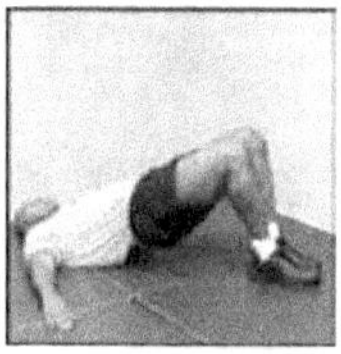

Back Bridge Position

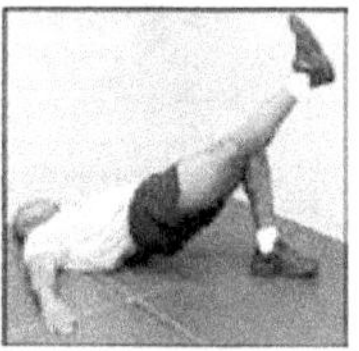

Right Leg Back Bridge

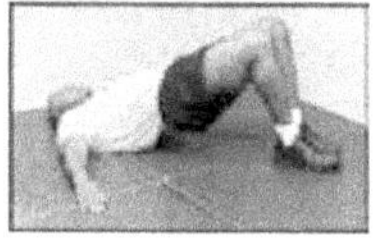

Back Bridge Position

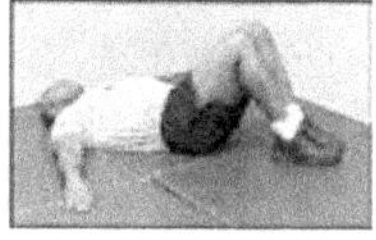

Starting Position

THE QUADRAPLEX

The Starting Position is on the hands and knees with the back flat.
Contract the abdominal muscles as described in the bent-leg raise.
Without rotating the trunk or sagging/arching the spine, straighten the
left leg to the rear and the right arm to the front. Hold five seconds.
Alternate the arm and leg movements on subsequent repetitions,
repeating for one minute. The key to this exercise is controlled lowering
and raising of the opposite arm/leg while keeping the rest of the
body still.

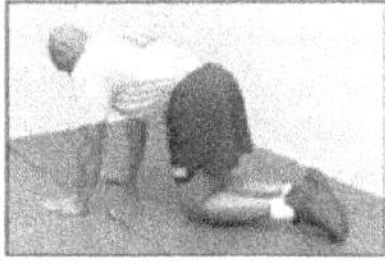

Starting Position

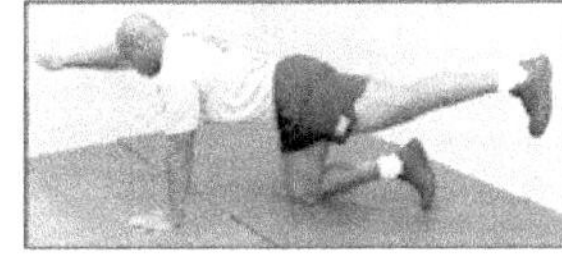

Right Quadraplex

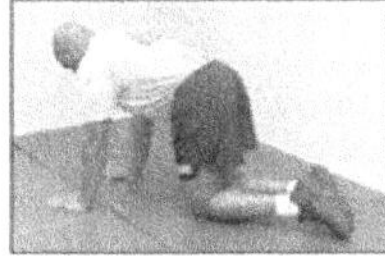

Starting Position

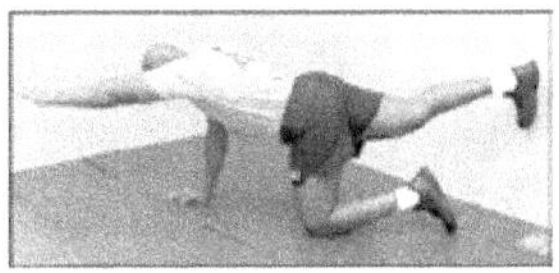

Left Quadraplex

The Hip Stability Drill

The Hip Stability Drill, like 4 for the Core, is designed to three-dimensionally train the hip and upper thigh areas, developing the basic strength and mobility needed for stability to perform functional movements. The Hip Stability Drill should be performed immediately after 4 for the Core. The Hip Stability Drill and 4 for the Core may performed outside of regular sessions as supplemental training.

Hip Stability Drill
Exercise 1: The Lateral Leg Raise
(5 repetitions on each side)

Purpose:	This exercise strengthens lateral hip and upper leg muscles.
Starting Position 1:	Lay on your right side with your legs extended straight to the side and feet together with toes pointing straight ahead. Support your upper body with your right elbow. Your elbow is bent at 90-degrees, your upper arm is perpendicular to the ground and your right hand makes a fist vertical to the ground.
Starting Position 2:	Lay on your left side with your legs extended straight to the side and feet together with toes pointing straight ahead. Support your upper body with your left elbow. Your elbow is bent at 90-degrees, your upper arm is perpendicular to the ground and your left hand makes a fist vertical to the ground.
Cadence:	SLOW.
Count:	1. Raise the bottom foot so the top foot is 6-8 inches above the ground.
	2 Return to the Starting Position.
	3. Raise the bottom foot so the top foot is 6-8 inches above the ground.
	4. Return to the Starting Position.

Left Lateral Leg Raise

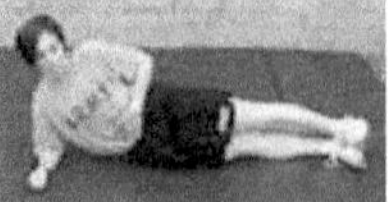

Starting Position

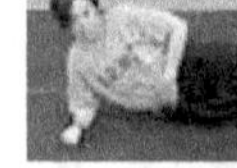

Count 1

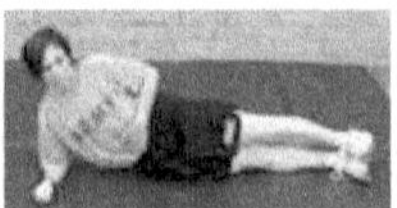

Count 2

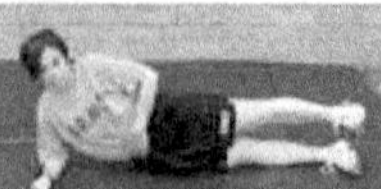

Count 3

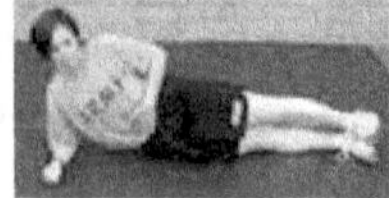

Count 4

Right Lateral Leg Raise

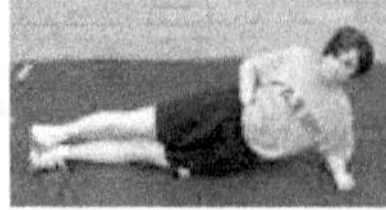

Starting Position

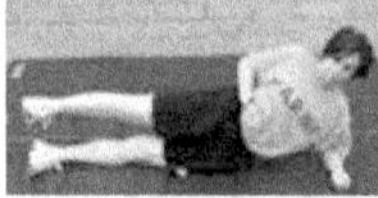

Count 1

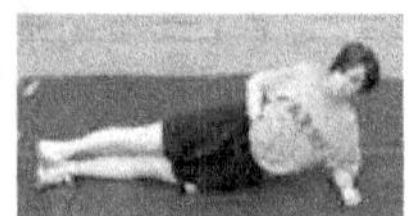

Count 2

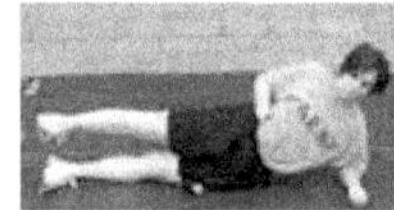

Count 3

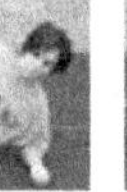

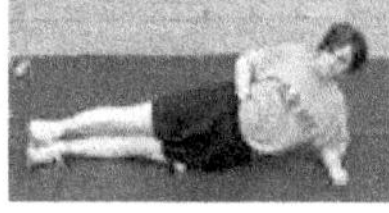

Count 4

Check Points:

- ❏ Face to the front of the formation, maintaining a generally straight line with the body.
- ❏ On Counts 1 and 3, keep the knee of the raised leg straight and the foot pointing forward. The top leg raises no more than 6-8 inches above the ground.
- ❏ Place the top hand over the stomach throughout the exercise.

Precautions: N/A.

Hip Stability Drill
Exercise 2: The Medial Leg Raise
(5 repetitions on each side)

Purpose:	This exercise strengthens the inner thigh and hip muscles.
Starting Position 1:	Lay on your left side with your legs extended straight to the side and feet together with toes pointing straight ahead. Support your upper body with your left elbow. Your elbow is bent at 90-degrees, your upper arm is perpendicular to the ground and your left hand makes a fist vertical to the ground.
Starting Position 2:	Lay on your right side with your legs extended straight to the side and feet together with toes pointing straight ahead. Support your upper body with your right elbow. Your elbow is bent at 90-degrees, your upper arm is perpendicular to the ground and your right hand makes a fist vertical to the ground.
Cadence:	SLOW.
Count:	1. Raise the top leg so the top foot is 6-8 inches above the ground.
	2 Return to the Starting Position.
	3. Raise the top leg so the top foot is 6-8 inches above the ground.
	4. Return to the Starting Position.

Left Medial Leg Raise

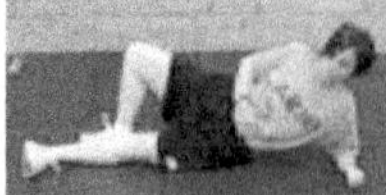

Starting Position

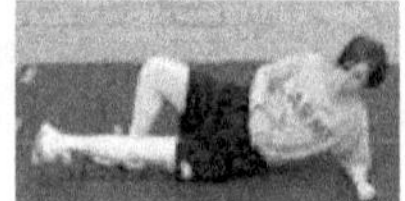

Count 1

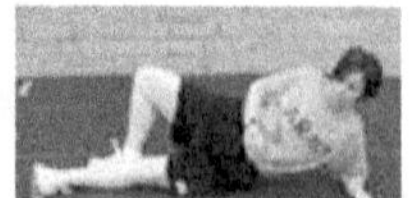

Count 2

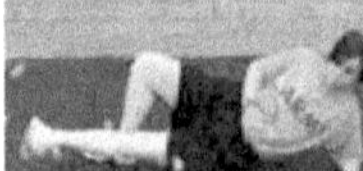

Count 3

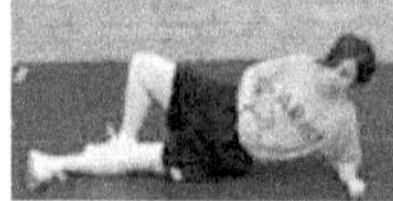

Count 4

Right Medial Leg Raise

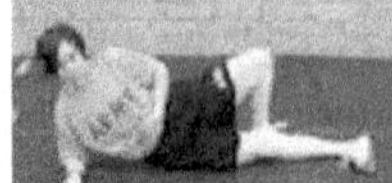

Starting Position

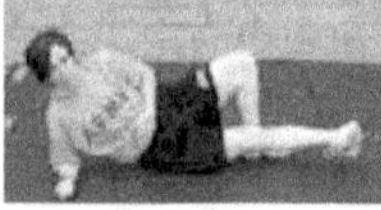

Count 1

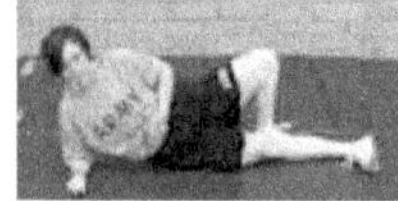

Count 2

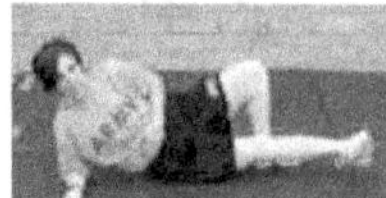

Count 3

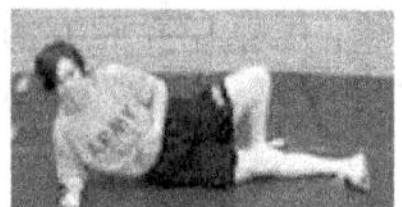

Count 4

Check Points:

- ❏ Keep the hips facing forward and the body in a generally straight line.
- ❏ Keep the toes facing forward on the bottom leg.
- ❏ Place the top hand over the stomach throughout the exercise.
- ❏ Do not raise the bottom foot higher than 6-8 inches above the ground.

Precautions: N/A.

Hip Stability Drill
Exercise 3: The Lateral Bent-leg Raise
(5 repetitions on each side)

Purpose:	This exercise strengthens hip rotator muscles.
Starting Position 1:	Lay on your right side with your legs bent at 90-degrees and feet together with toes pointing straight ahead. Support your upper body with your right elbow. Your elbow is bent at 90-degrees, your upper arm is perpendicular to the ground and your right hand makes a fist vertical to the ground.
Starting Position 2:	Lay on your left side with your legs bent at 90-degrees and feet together with toes pointing straight ahead. Support your upper body with your left elbow. Your elbow is bent at 90-degrees, your upper arm is perpendicular to the ground and your left hand makes a fist vertical to the ground.
Cadence:	SLOW.
Count:	1. Raise the top leg approximately 12 inches above the ground, keeping the feet together.
	2. Return to the Starting Position.
	3. Raise the top leg approximately 12 inches above the ground, keeping the feet together.
	4. Return to the Starting Position.

Right Lateral Bent-leg Raise

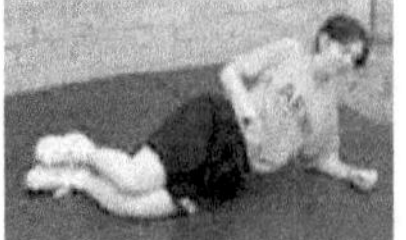

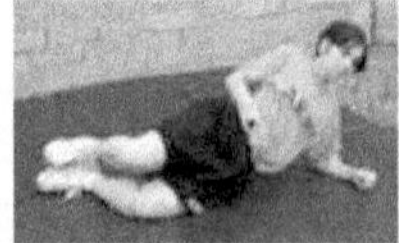

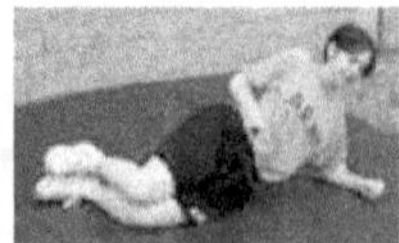

| Starting Position | Count 1 | Count 2 |

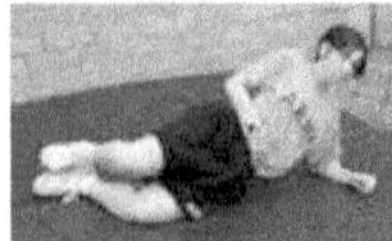

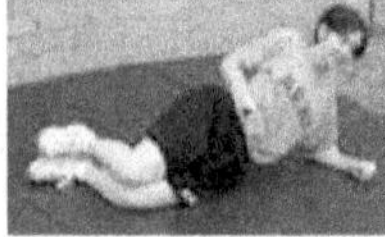

| Count 3 | Count 4 |

Left Lateral Bent-leg Raise

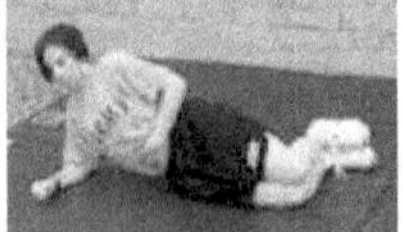

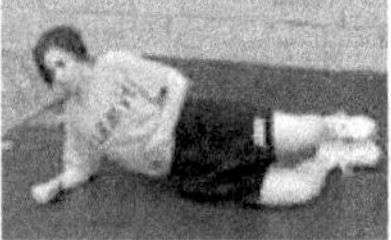

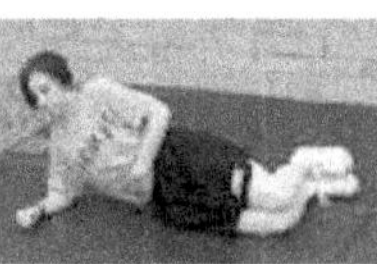

| Starting Position | Count 1 | Count 2 |

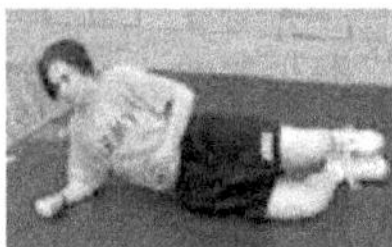

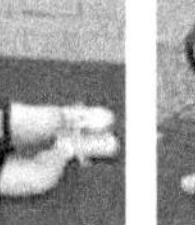

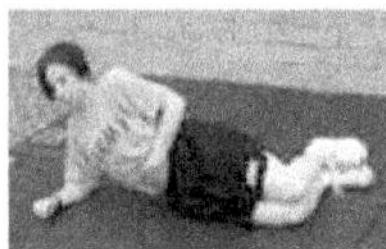

| Count 3 | Count 4 |

Check Points:

❑ Face to the front of the formation, maintaining a generally straight line with the body, from the knees to the torso.
❑ Keep the feet together throughout the exercise.
❑ Place the top hand over the stomach throughout the exercise.

Precautions: N/A.

Hip Stability Drill
Exercise 4: The Single-leg Tuck
(5 repetitions on each side)

Purpose: This exercise strengthens the hip flexors, lateral hip and upper leg muscles.

Starting Position 1: Lay on your right side with your legs extended straight to the side, with the left leg 6-8 inches above the ground and toes pointing straight ahead. Support your upper body with your right elbow. Your elbow is bent at 90-degrees, your upper arm is perpendicular to the ground and your right hand makes a fist vertical to the ground.

Starting Position 2: Lay on your left side with your legs extended straight to the side, with the right leg 6-8 inches above the ground and toes pointing straight ahead. Support your upper body with your left elbow. Your elbow is bent at 90-degrees, your upper arm is perpendicular to the ground and your left hand makes a fist vertical to the ground.

Cadence: SLOW.

Count:
1. Bring the thigh of the top leg toward the chest, bending the knee at 90-degrees.
2. Return to the Starting Position.
3. Bring the thigh of the top leg toward the chest, bending the knee at 90-degrees.
4. Return to the Starting Position.

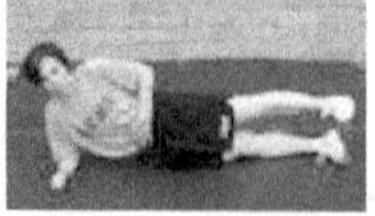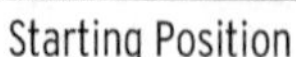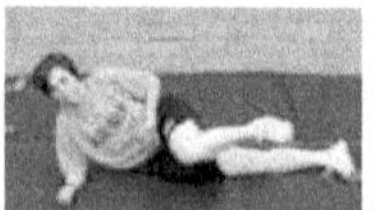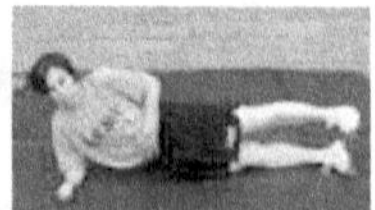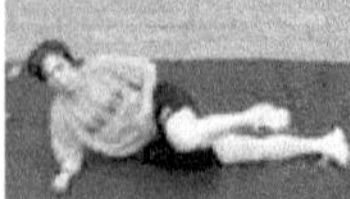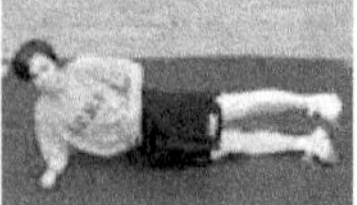

Left Single-leg Tuck

Starting Position	Count 1	Count 2

Count 3	Count 4

Right Single-leg Tuck

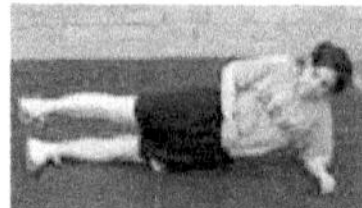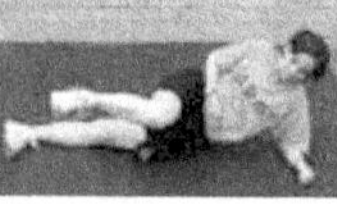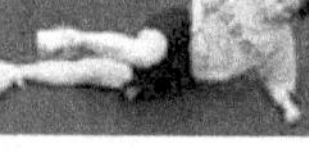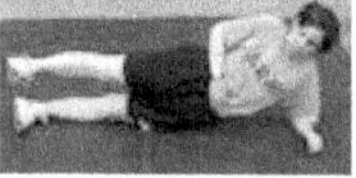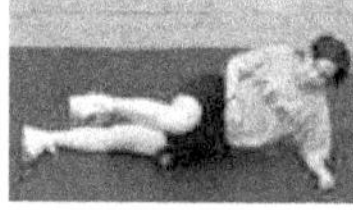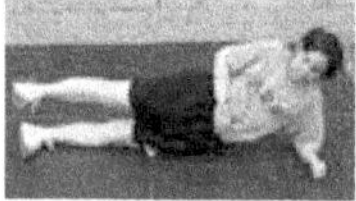

Starting Position	Count 1	Count 2

Count 3	Count 4

Check Points:

- ❑ Face to the front of the formation, maintaining a generally straight line with the body.
- ❑ The top foot remains 6-8 inches above the ground throughout the exercise.
- ❑ Place the top hand over the stomach throughout the exercise.

Precautions: N/A.

Hip Stability Drill
Exercise 5: The Single-leg Over
(hold for 20 seconds on each side)

Purpose:	This exercise develops flexibility of the hips and lower back muscles.
Starting Position:	Supine position with arms sideward, palms down.
Exercise Position 1:	On the command, **"Ready, STRETCH,"** turn the body to right, bend the left knee to 90-degrees over the right leg and grasp the outside of the left knee with the right hand and pull toward the right. Hold this position for 20 seconds.
Starting Position:	On the command, **"Starting Position, MOVE,"** assume the Starting Position.
Exercise Position 2:	On the command, **"Ready, STRETCH,"** turn the body to left, bend the right knee to 90-degrees over the left leg and grasp the outside of the right knee with the left hand and pull toward the left. Hold this position for 20 seconds.
Starting Position:	On the command, **"Starting Position, MOVE,"** assume the Starting Position.

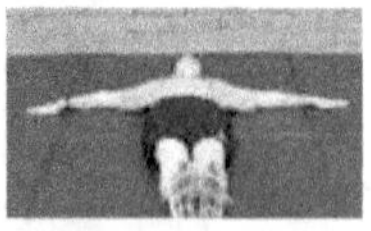

Starting Position

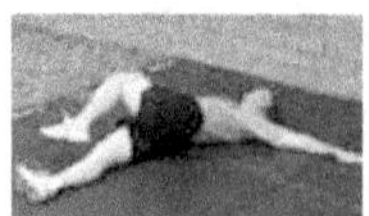

Exercise Position 1

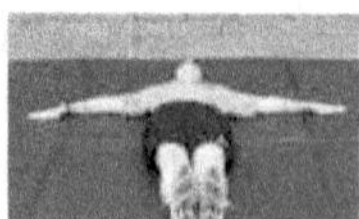

Starting Position

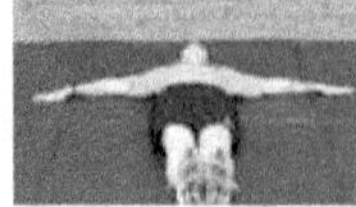

Starting Position

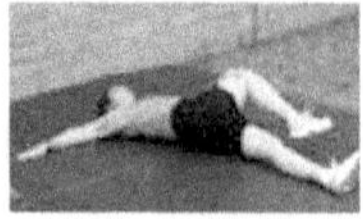

Exercise Position 2

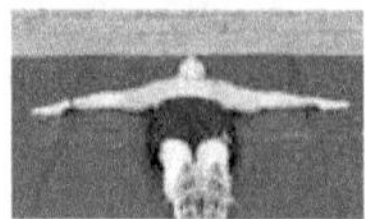

Starting Position

Check Points:

- ❏ At the Starting Position, the arms are directed to the sides at 90-degrees to the trunk; the fingers and thumbs are extended and joined.
- ❏ In Exercise Position 1, keep the left shoulder, arm and hand on the ground.
- ❏ In Exercise Position 2, keep the right shoulder, arm and hand on the ground.
- ❏ Head remains on the ground throughout the exercise.

Precautions: N/A.

Conditioning Drill 1
Exercise 1: The Bend and Reach

Purpose:	This exercise develops the ability to squat and reach through the legs. It also serves to prepare the spine and extremities for more vigorous movements, moving the hips and spine through full flexion.
Starting Position:	Straddle stance with arms overhead.
Cadence:	SLOW.
Count:	1. Squat with the heels flat as the spine rounds forward to allow the straight arms to reach as far as possible between the legs. 2. Return to the Starting Position. 3. Repeat Count 1. 4. Return to the Starting Position.

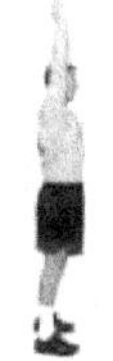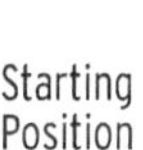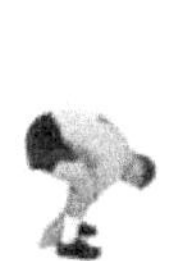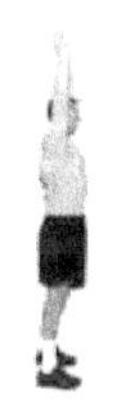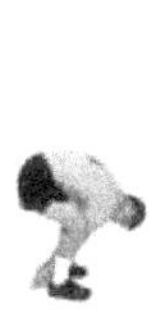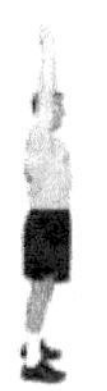

Starting Position	Count 1	Count 2	Count 3	Count 4

Check Points:

- From the Starting Position, ensure that Soldiers have their hips set, their abdominals tight, and their arms fully extended overhead.
- The neck flexes to allow the gaze to the rear. This brings the head in line with the bend of the trunk.
- The heels and feet remain flat on the ground.
- On Counts 2 and 4, do not go past the Starting Position.

Precautions: This exercise is always performed at a slow cadence.
To protect the back, move into the Count 1 position in a slow, controlled manner. Do not bounce into or out of this position in a ballistic manner, as this may place an excessive load on the back.

Conditioning Drill 1
Exercise 2: The Rear Lunge

Purpose:	This exercise promotes balance, opens up the hip and trunk on the side of the lunge and develops leg strength.
Starting Position:	Straddle stance with hands on hips.
Cadence:	SLOW.
Count:	1. Take an exaggerated step backward with the left leg, touching down with the ball of the foot.
	2. Return to the Starting Position.
	3. Repeat Count 1 with the right leg.
	4. Return to the Starting Position.

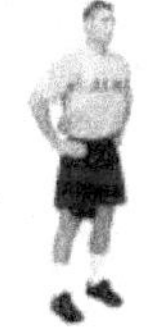 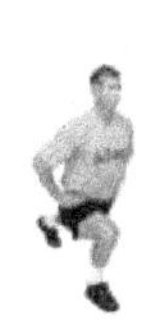 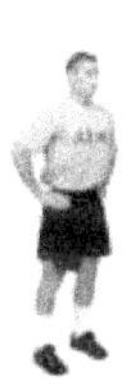 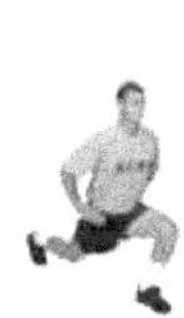 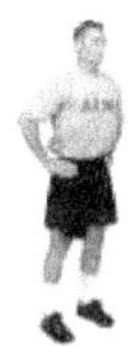

Starting Position   Count 1   Count 2   Count 3   Count 4

Check Points:

- ❑ Maintain straightness of the back by keeping the abdominal muscles tight throughout the motion.
- ❑ After the foot touches down, allow the body to continue to lower. This promotes flexibility of the hip and trunk.
- ❑ On Counts 1 and 3, step straight to the rear, keeping the feet directed forward. When viewed from the front, the feet maintain their distance apart both at the Starting Position and at the end of Counts 1 and 3.
- ❑ Keep the rear leg as straight as possible but not locked.

Precautions: This exercise is always performed at a slow cadence.
On Counts 1 and 3, move into position in a slow, controlled manner.
If the cadence is too fast, it will be difficult to go through a full range
of motion.

Conditioning Drill 1
Exercise 3: The High Jumper

Purpose: This exercise reinforces correct jumping and landing, stimulates balance and coordination, and develops explosive strength.

Starting Position: Forward-leaning stance.

Cadence: MODERATE.

Count:

1. Swing arms forward and jump a few inches.
2. Swing arms backward and jump a few inches.
3. Swing arms forward and vigorously over head while jumping forcefully.
4. Repeat Count 2. On the last repetition, return to the Starting Position.

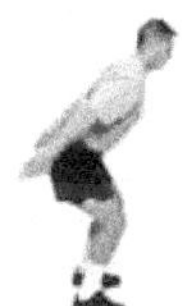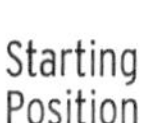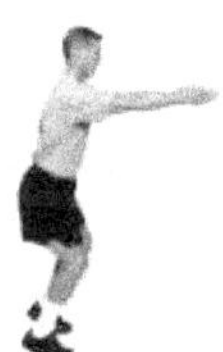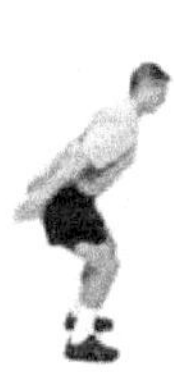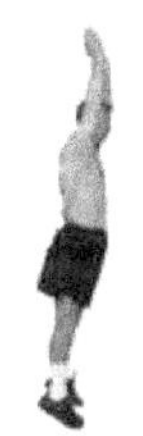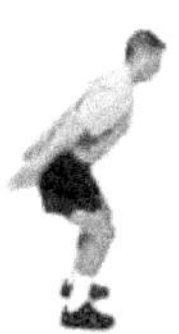

Starting Position	Count 1	Count 2	Count 3	Count 4

Check Points:

- ❏ At the Starting Position, the shoulders, the knees, and the balls of the feet should form a straight vertical line.
- ❏ On Count 1, the arms are parallel to the ground.
- ❏ On Count 3, the arms should be extended fully overhead. The trunk and legs should also be in line.
- ❏ On each landing, the feet should be directed forward and maintained at shoulder distance apart. The landing should be "soft" and proceed from balls of the feet to the heels. The vertical line from the shoulders through the knees to the balls of the feet should be demonstrated on each landing.

Precautions: N/A.

Conditioning Drill 1
Exercise 4: The Rower

Purpose: This exercise improves the ability to move in and out of the supine position to a seated posture. It coordinates the action of the trunk and extremities while challenging the abdominal muscles.

Starting Position: Supine position, arms overhead, feet together and pointing upward. The chin is tucked, and the head is one to two inches above the ground. Arms are shoulder width, palms facing inward with fingers and thumbs extended and joined.

Cadence: SLOW.

Count:
1. Sit up while swinging arms forward and bending at the hip and knees. At the end of the motion, the arms will be parallel to ground, palms facing inward.
2. Return to the Starting Position.
3. Repeat Count 1.
4. Return to the Starting Position.

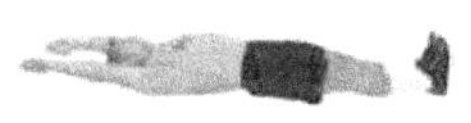

Starting
Position

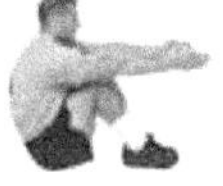

Count 1

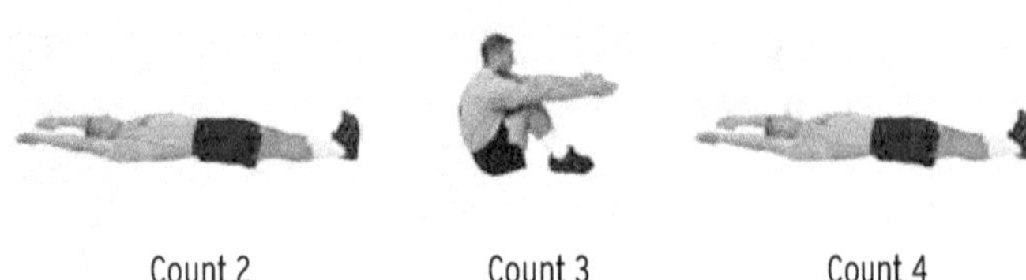

Count 2   Count 3   Count 4

Check Points:

❑ At the Starting Position, the lower back must not be arched excessively off the ground. To prevent this, tighten the abdominal muscles to tilt the pelvis and lower back toward the ground.

❑ At the end of Counts 1 and 3, the feet are flat and pulled near the buttocks. The legs stay together throughout the exercise and the arms are parallel to the ground.

Precautions: This exercise is always performed at a slow cadence. Do not arch the back to assume Counts 1 and 3.

Conditioning Drill 1
Exercise 5: The Squat Bender

Purpose: This exercise develops strength, endurance and flexibility of the lower back and lower extremities.

Starting Position: Straddle stance with hands on hips.

Cadence: SLOW.

Count:
1. Squat while leaning slightly forward at the waist with the head up and extend the arms to the front, with arms parallel to the ground and palms facing inward.
2. Return to the Starting Position.
3. Bend forward and reach toward the ground with both arms extended and palms inward.
4. Return to the Starting Position.

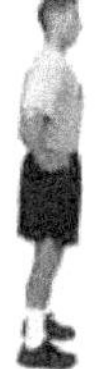

Starting
Position

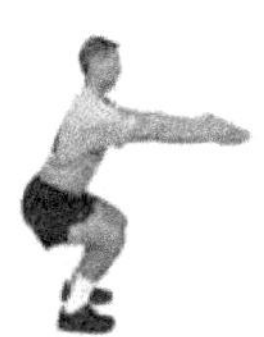

Count 1

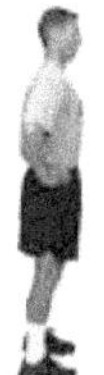

Count 2

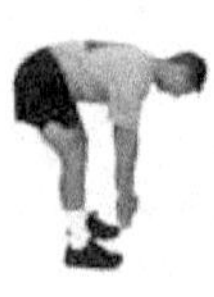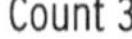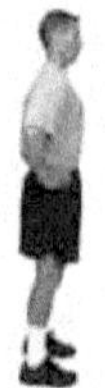

Count 3

Count 4

Check Points:

- ❏ At the end of Count 1, the shoulders, knees and balls of the feet should be aligned. The heels remain on the ground and the back is straight.
- ❏ On Count 3, round the back slightly while bending forward, keeping the head aligned with the spine and the knees slightly bent.

Precautions: This exercise is always performed at a slow cadence. Allowing the knees to go beyond the toes on Count 1 increases stress to the knees.

Conditioning Drill 1
Exercise 6: The Windmill

Purpose:	This exercise develops the ability to safely bend and rotate the trunk. It conditions the muscles of the trunk, legs, and shoulders.
Starting Position:	Straddle stance with arms sideward, palms facing down.
Cadence:	SLOW.

Count:

1. Bend the hips and knees while rotating to the left. Reach down and touch the outside of the left foot with the right hand and look toward the rear. The left arm is pulled rearward to maintain a straight line with the right arm.
2. Return to the Starting Position.
3. Repeat Count 1 to the right.
4. Return to the Starting Position.

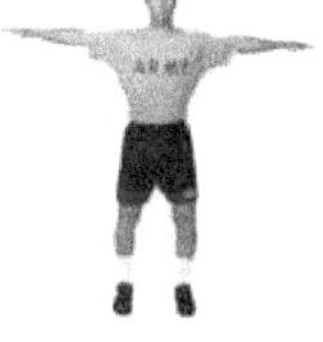

Starting
Position

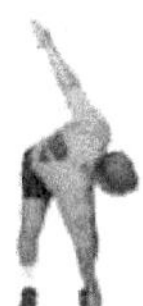

Count 1

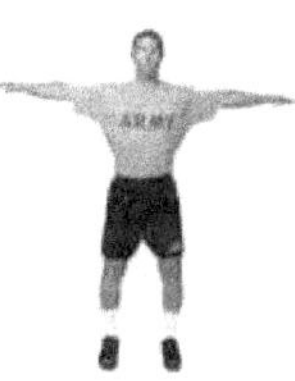

Count 2

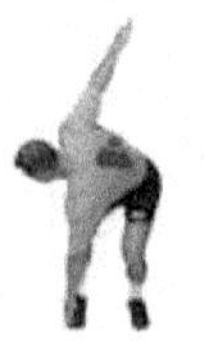
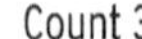
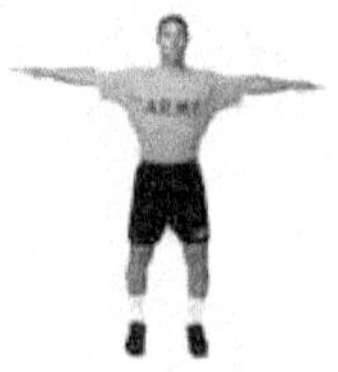

Count 3   Count 4

Check Points:

❑ From the Starting Position, feet are straight ahead, arms parallel to the ground, hips set, and abdominals tight.

❑ On Counts 1 and 3, ensure that the knees bend during the rotation. Head and eyes are directed to the left foot on Count 1 and the right foot on Count 3.

Precautions: This exercise is always performed at a slow cadence.

Conditioning Drill 1
Exercise 7: The Forward Lunge

Purpose:	This exercise promotes balance and develops leg strength.
Starting Position:	Straddle stance with hands on hips.
Cadence:	SLOW.
Count:	1. Take a step forward with the left leg, allowing the left knee to bend until the thigh is parallel to the ground. Lean slightly forward, keeping the back straight.
	2. Return to the Starting Position.
	3. Repeat Count 1 with the right leg.
	4. Return to the Starting Position.

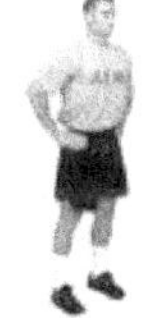

Starting
Position

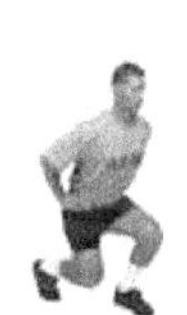

Count 1

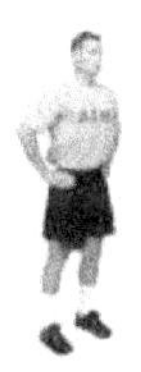

Count 2

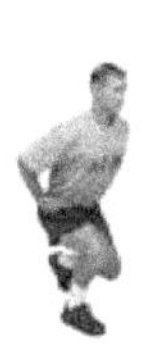

Count 3

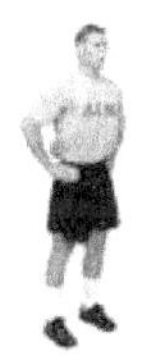

Count 4

Check Points:

❑ Keep the abdominal muscles tight throughout the motion.
❑ On Counts 1 and 3, step straight forward, keeping the feet directed
forward. When viewed from the front, the feet maintain
their distance apart both at the Starting Position and at the end
of Counts 1 and 3.
❑ On Counts 1 and 3, the rear knee may bend naturally but do not touch
the ground. The heel of the rear foot should be off the ground.

Precautions: This exercise is always performed at a slow cadence.
On Counts 1 and 3, move into position in a controlled manner. Spring off
of the forward leg to return to the Starting Position. This avoids jerking
the trunk to create momentum.

Conditioning Drill 1
Exercise 8: The Prone Row

Purpose: This exercise develops strength of the back and shoulders.

Starting Position: Prone position with the arms overhead, palms down one to two inches off the ground and toes pointed to the rear.

Cadence: SLOW.

Count:
1. Raise the head and chest slightly while lifting the arms and pulling them rearward. Hands make fists as they move toward the shoulders.
2. Return to the Starting Position.
3. Repeat Count 1.
4. Return to the Starting Position.

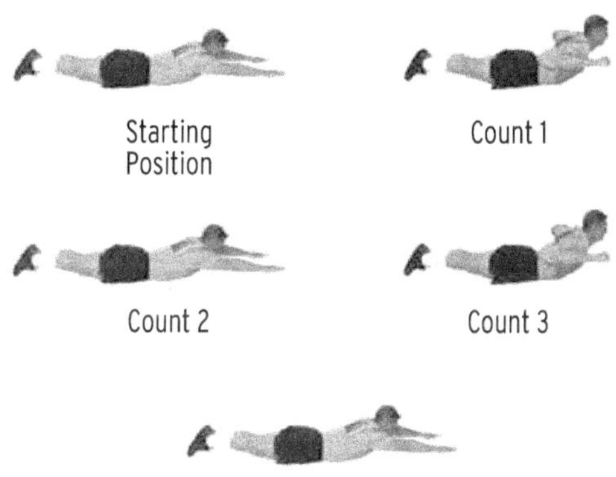

Starting
Position

Count 1

Count 2

Count 3

Count 4

Check Points:

- ❑ At the Starting Position, the abdominal muscles are tight and the head is in line with the spine.
- ❑ On Counts 1 and 3, the forearms are parallel to the ground and slightly higher than the trunk.
- ❑ On Counts 1 and 3, the head is raised to look forward but not skyward.
- ❑ Throughout the exercise, the legs and toes remain in contact with the ground.

Precautions: This exercise is always performed at a slow cadence. Prevent over-arching of the back by maintaining contractions of the abdominal and buttocks muscles throughout the exercise.

Conditioning Drill 1
Exercise 9: The Bent-leg Body Twist

Purpose: This exercise strengthens trunk muscles and promotes control of trunk rotation.

Starting Position: Supine position with the hips and knees bent to 90-degrees, arms sideward, palms down with fingers spread. Legs and feet are together.

Cadence: SLOW.

Count:
1. Rotate the legs to the left while keeping the upper back and arms in place.
2. Return to the Starting Position.
3. Repeat Count 1 to the right.
4. Return to the Starting Position.

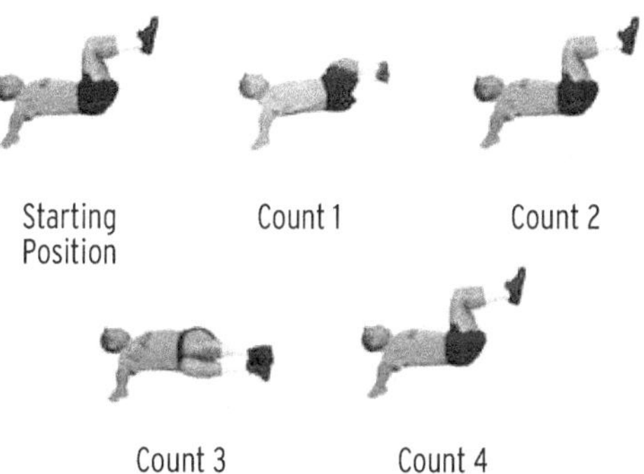

Starting Position

Count 1

Count 2

Count 3

Count 4

Check Points:

- ❏ Tighten the abdominal muscles in the Starting Position and maintain this contraction throughout the exercise.
- ❏ The head should be off the ground with the chin slightly tucked.
- ❏ Ensure that the hips and knees maintain 90-degree angles.
- ❏ Keep the feet and knees together throughout the exercise.
- ❏ Attempt to rotate the legs to about 8-10 inches off the ground. The opposite shoulder must remain in contact with the ground.

Precautions: This exercise is always performed at a slow cadence. Do not rotate the legs to a point beyond which they can no longer maintain contact with the ground with the opposite arm and shoulder.

Conditioning Drill 1
Exercise 10: The Push-up

Purpose: This exercise strengthens the muscles of the chest, shoulders, arms and trunk.

Starting Position: Front leaning rest position.

Cadence: MODERATE.

Count:
1. Bend the elbows, lowering the body until the upper arms are parallel with the ground.
2. Return to the Starting Position.
3. Repeat Count 1.
4. Return to the Starting Position.

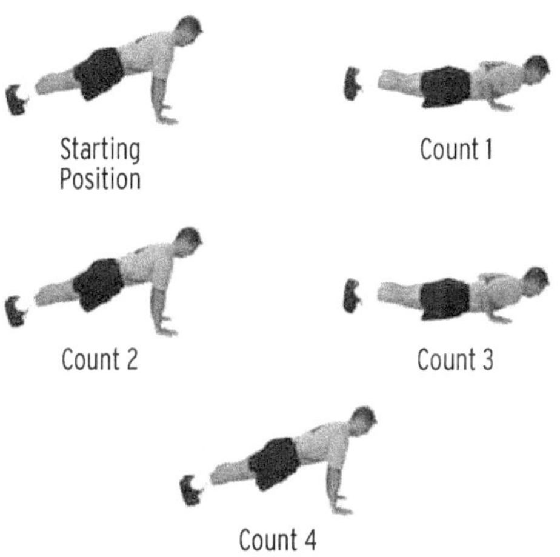

Starting
Position

Count 1

Count 2

Count 3

Count 4

Check Points:

- ❏ The hands are directly below the shoulders with fingers spread (middle fingers point straight ahead).
- ❏ On Counts 1 and 3 the upper arms stay close to the trunk, elbows pointing rearward.
- ❏ On Counts 2 and 4 the elbows straighten but do not lock.
- ❏ The trunk should not sag. To prevent this, tighten the abdominal muscles while in the Starting Position and maintain this contraction throughout the exercise.

Precautions: N/A.

Variation: Soldiers should assume the six-point stance on their knees when unable to perform repetitions correctly to cadence.

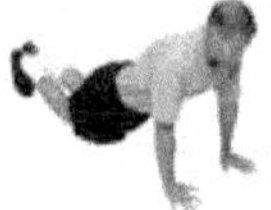 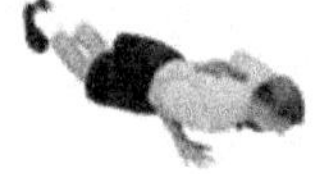

The Military Movement Drill
Exercise 1: Verticals

Purpose: This exercise helps to develop proper running form.

Starting Position: Staggered stance.

Movement: Bring the hips quickly to 90-degrees of bend without raising the knees above waist level. Ground contact should be primarily with the balls of the feet. When the left leg is forward, the right arm swings forward and the left arm swings to the rear. When the right leg is forward, the left arm swings forward and the right arm swings to the rear.

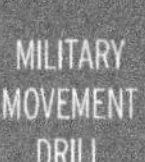

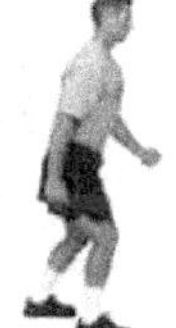 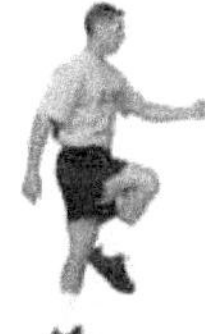 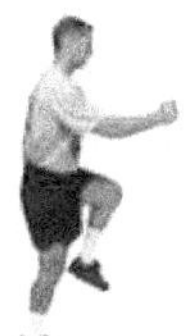 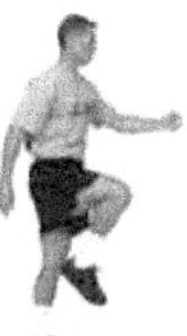 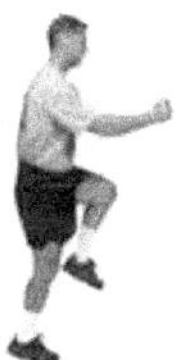

Starting Position ⟶

Check Points:

- ❑ Arm swing is strong and smooth with the forward arm at 90-degrees and the rearward arm relatively straight.
- ❑ Arm swing is from front to rear, not side to side, with the upper part of the forward arm reaching parallel to the ground as it swings to the front.
- ❑ Keep a tall stance with a stable, upright trunk. The back remains perpendicular to the ground. There should not be any back swing of the legs.

Precautions: N/A.

The Military Movement Drill
Exercise 2: Laterals

Purpose: This exercise develops the ability to move laterally.

Starting Position: Straddle stance, slightly crouched, with the back straight, arms at the side with elbows bent at 90-degrees and palms facing forward. Face perpendicular to the direction of movement.

Movement: Step to the side by rising slightly and bringing the trailing leg to the lead leg. Quickly hop to the side and land back in the crouch with the feet shoulder width apart. Always face the same direction so that the first 25 yards is moving to the left and the second 25 yards is moving to the right.

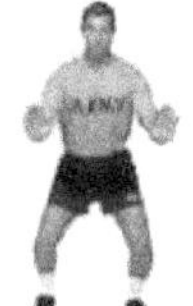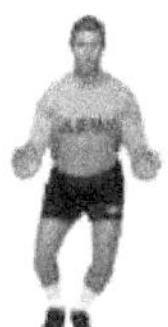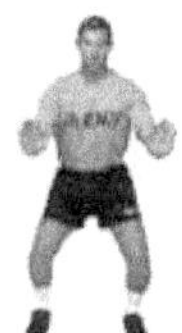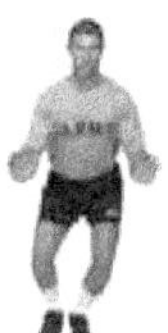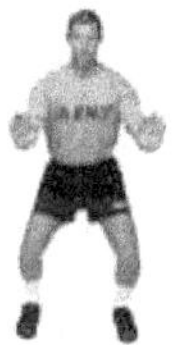

Starting Position →

Check Points:

- ❏ Pick the feet up with each step. Avoid dragging the feet along the ground.
- ❏ Crouch slightly while keeping the back straight.
- ❏ Avoid hitting the feet and ankles together on each step.
- ❏ Rank leaders will face their rank throughout the exercise.

Precautions: N/A.

Variation: Soldiers may perform this exercise holding a weapon at port arms.

The Military Movement Drill
Exercise 3: The Shuttle Sprint

Purpose: This exercise develops anaerobic endurance, leg speed, and agility.

Starting Position: Staggered stance.

Movement: Run quickly to the 25-yard mark. Turn clockwise while planting the left foot and bending and squatting to touch the ground with the left hand. Run quickly back to the starting line and plant the right foot, turn counterclockwise and touch the ground with the right hand. Run back to the 25-yard mark gradually accelerating to near maximum speed.

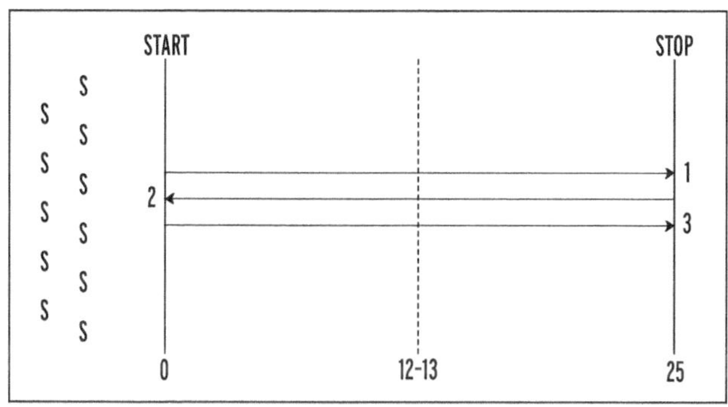

Check Points:

- ❑ Soldiers should slow their movement before planting feet and changing direction.
- ❑ Soldiers should squat while bending the trunk when reaching to touch the ground as they change direction.
- ❑ Soldiers touch the ground with their left hand on the first turn, then with their right hand on the second turn.
- ❑ Accelerate to near maximum speed during the last 25-yard interval.

Precautions: Soldiers should use caution when performing this exercise on wet terrain.

The Stretch Drill
Exercise 1: The Overhead Arm Pull

Purpose: This exercise develops flexibility of the arms, shoulders, and trunk muscles.

Starting Position: Straddle stance with hands on hips.

- On the command, **"Ready, STRETCH,"** raise the left arm overhead and place the left hand behind the head. Grasp above the left elbow with the right hand and pull to the right, leaning the body to the right. Hold this position for 20 seconds.
- On the command, **"Starting Position, MOVE,"** assume the Starting Position.
- On the command, **"Change Position, Ready, STRETCH,"** raise the right arm overhead and place the right hand behind the head. Grasp above the right elbow with the left hand and pull to the left, leaning the body to the left. Hold this position for 20 seconds.
- On the command, **"Starting Position, MOVE,"** return to the Starting Position.

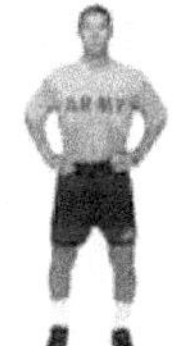

Starting Position

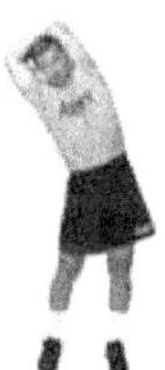

Position 1

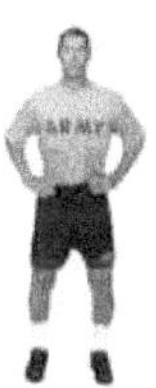

Starting Position

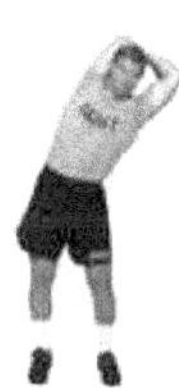

Position 2

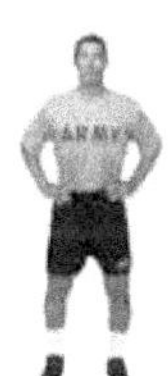

Starting Position

Check Points:

❑ Throughout the exercise, keep the hips set and the abdominals tight.

❑ In Positions 1 and 2, lean the body straight to the side, not to the front or back.

Precautions: N/A.

The Stretch Drill
Exercise 2: The Rear Lunge

Purpose: This exercise develops flexibility of the hip flexors and trunk muscles.

Starting Position: Straddle stance with hands on hips.

- On the command, **"Ready, STRETCH,"** take an exaggerated step backward with the left leg, touching down with the ball of the foot. This is the same position as Count 1 of The Rear Lunge in Conditioning Drill 1. Hold this position for 20 seconds.
- On the command, **"Starting Position, MOVE,"** assume the Starting Position.
- On the command, **"Change Position, Ready, STRETCH,"** take an exaggerated step backward with the right leg, touching down with the ball of the foot. This is the same position as Count 3 of The Rear Lunge in Conditioning Drill 1. Hold this position for 20 seconds.
- On the command, **"Starting Position, MOVE,"** return to the Starting Position.

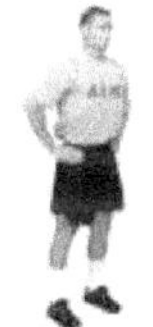

Starting
Position

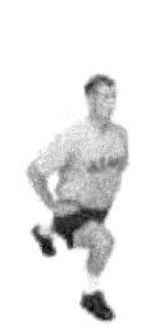

Position 1

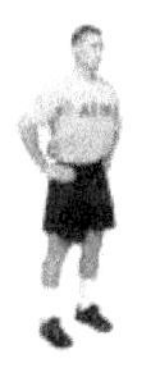

Starting
Position

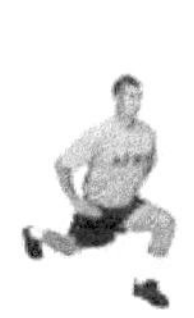

Position 2

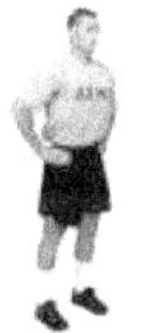

Starting
Position

Check Points:

- ❏ Maintain straightness of the back by keeping the abdominal muscles tight throughout the motion.
- ❏ After the foot touches down on Positions 1 and 2, allow the body to continue to lower.
- ❏ Lunge and step in a straight line, keeping the feet directed forward. Viewed from the front, the feet are shoulder width apart, both at the Starting Position, and at the end of Positions 1 and 2.
- ❏ Keep the forward knee over the ball of the foot on Positions 1 and 2.

Precautions: When lunging to the left or right do not let the knee move forward of the toes.

The Stretch Drill
Exercise 3: The Extend and Flex

Purpose: This exercise develops flexibility of the hip flexors, abdominals, hip (Position 1 - extend) and the low back, hamstrings, and calves (Position 2 - flex).

Starting Position: Front leaning rest position.

- On the command, **"Ready, STRETCH,"** lower the body, sagging in the middle, keeping the arms straight and look upward. Hold this position for 20 seconds.
- On the command, **"Starting Position, MOVE,"** assume the Starting Position.
- On the command, **"Change Position, Ready, STRETCH,"** slightly bend the knees and walk the hands back toward the legs. Straighten the legs and try to touch the ground with the heels. Keep the feet together and hold this position for 20 seconds.
- On the command, **"Starting Position, MOVE,"** return to the Starting Position.

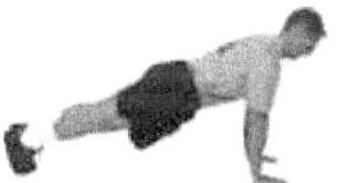

Starting
Position

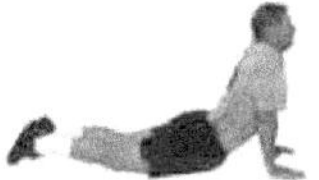

Position 1

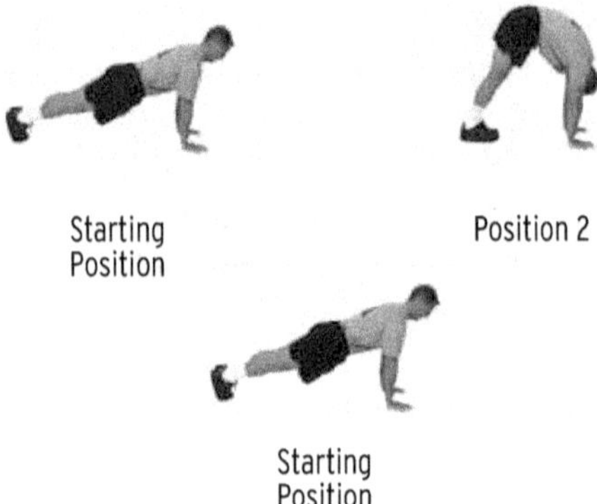

Check Points:

- ❏ In Position 1, the thighs and pelvis rest on the ground. Relax the back muscles while bearing the body weight through the straight arms. Toes point to the rear.
- ❏ In Position 2, the legs are straight and the arms are shoulder width apart, palms down on the ground.
- ❏ Feet are together throughout the exercise.

Precautions: N/A.

The Stretch Drill
Exercise 4: The Thigh Stretch

Purpose: This exercise develops flexibility of the front of the thigh and the hip flexor muscles.

Starting Position: Seated position, arms at sides and palms on the floor.

- On the command, **"Ready, STRETCH,"** roll onto the right side and place the right forearm on the ground, perpendicular to the chest. The right hand makes a fist on the ground with the thumb side up. Grasp the left ankle with the left hand and pull the left heel toward the buttocks and pull the entire leg rearward. Push the left thigh further to the rear with the bottom of the right foot. Hold this position for 20 seconds.
- On the command, **"Starting Position, MOVE,"** assume the Starting Position.
- On the command, **"Change Position, Ready, STRETCH,"** lay on the left side and place the left forearm on the ground, perpendicular to the chest. The left hand makes a fist on the ground with the thumb side up. Grasp the right ankle with the right hand and pull the right heel toward the buttocks and pull the entire leg rearward. Push the right thigh further to the rear with the bottom of the left foot. Hold this position for 20 seconds.
- On the command, **"Starting Position, MOVE,"** return to the Starting Position.

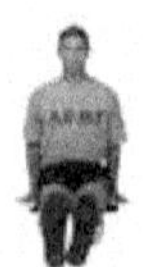

Starting
Position

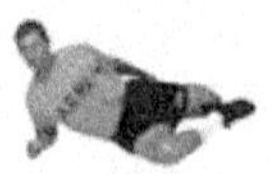

Position 1

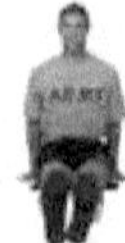

Starting
Position

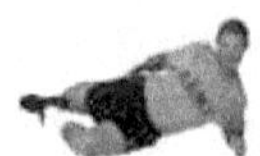

Position 2

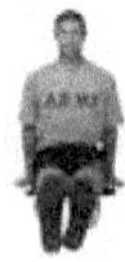

Starting
Position

Check Points:

❑ Keep the abdominal muscles tight throughout this stretch in order to
keep the trunk straight.
❑ Do not pull the heel forcefully to the buttock if there is discomfort in
the knee joint.

Precautions: N/A.

The Stretch Drill
Exercise 5: The Single-leg Over

Purpose: This exercise develops flexibility of the hips and lower back muscles.

Starting Position: Supine position with arms sideward, palms down.

- On the command, **"Ready, STRETCH,"** turn the body to the right, bend the left knee to 90-degrees over the right leg, and grasp the outside of the left knee with the right hand and pull toward the right. Hold this position for 20 seconds.
- On the command, **"Starting Position, MOVE,"** assume the Starting Position.
- On the command, **"Change Position, Ready, STRETCH,"** turn the body to the left, bend the right knee to 90-degrees over the left leg, and grasp the outside of the right knee with the left hand and pull toward the left. Hold this position for 20 seconds.
- On the command, **"Starting Position, MOVE,"** return to the Starting Position.

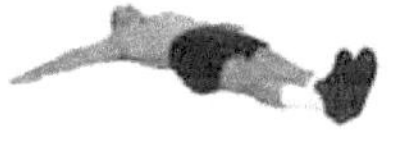

Starting
Position

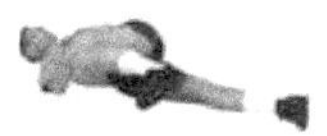

Position 1

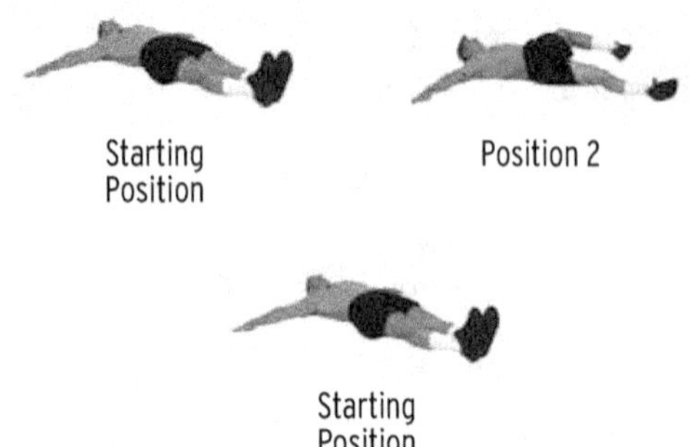

Check Points:

❏ At the Starting Position, the arms are directed to the sides at
   90-degrees to the trunk, the fingers and thumbs are extended
   and joined.
❏ In Position 1, keep the left shoulder, arm, and hand on the ground.
❏ In Position 2, keep the right shoulder, arm, and hand on the ground.

Precautions: N/A.

Conditioning Drill 2
Exercise 1: The Push-up

Purpose:	This exercise strengthens the muscles of the chest, shoulders, arms and trunk.
Starting Position:	Front leaning rest position.
Cadence:	MODERATE.
Count:	1. Bend the elbows, lowering the body until the upper arms are parallel with the ground. 2. Return to the Starting Position. 3. Repeat Count 1. 4. Return to the Starting Position.

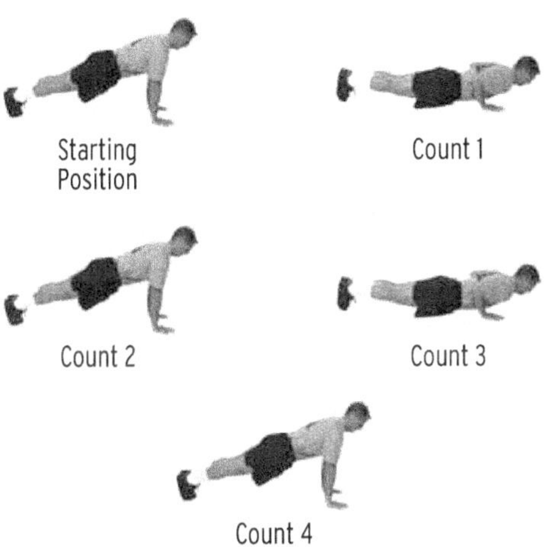

Starting Position

Count 1

Count 2

Count 3

Count 4

Check Points:

- ❑ The hands are directly below the shoulders with fingers spread (middle fingers point straight ahead).
- ❑ On Counts 1 and 3 the upper arms stay close to the trunk, elbows pointing rearward.
- ❑ On Counts 2 and 4 the elbows straighten but do not lock.
- ❑ The trunk should not sag. To prevent this, tighten the abdominal muscles while in the Starting Position and maintain this contraction throughout the exercise.

Precautions: N/A.

Variation: Soldiers should assume the six-point stance on their knees when unable to perform repetitions correctly to cadence.

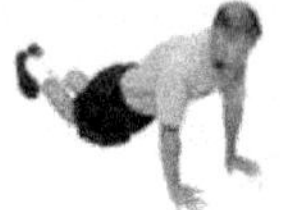 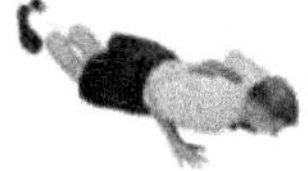

Conditioning Drill 2
Exercise 2: The Sit-up

Purpose: This exercise strengthens the abdominal and hip flexor muscles.

Starting Position: Supine position with hands behind head, fingers interlaced and knees bent at 90-degrees. Feet are together or up to 12 inches apart and flat on the ground. Hands are touching the ground.

Cadence: MODERATE.

Count:

1. Raise the upper body to the vertical position so that the base of the neck is above the base of the spine.
2. Return to the Starting Position in a controlled manner until the bottom of the shoulder blades touch the ground. The head and hands need not touch the ground.
3. Repeat Count 1.
4. Repeat Count 2 and return to the Starting Position at the completion of the final repetition.

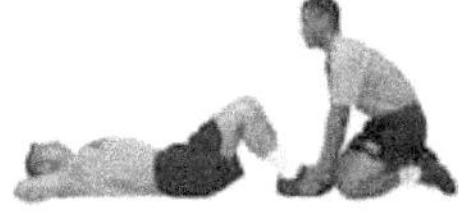

Starting Position

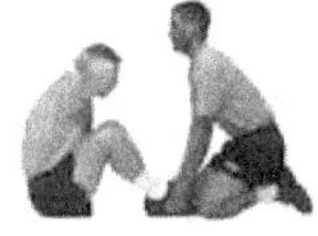

Count 1

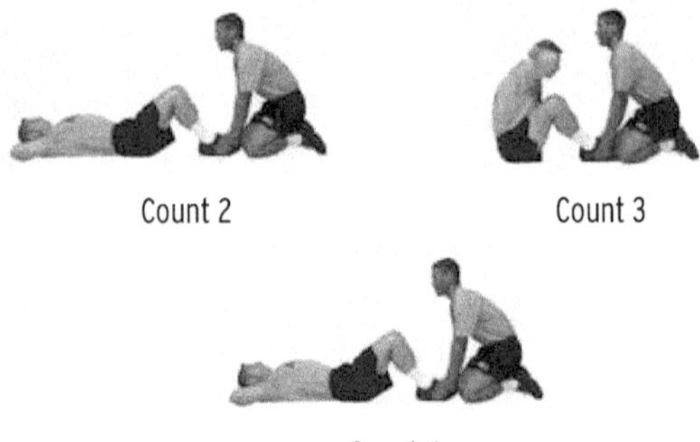

Count 2

Count 3

Count 4

Check Points:

- ❏ The hands are behind the head with the fingers interlaced.
- ❏ Feet are together or up to 12 inches apart and both heels must remain in contact with the ground throughout the exercise.
- ❏ On Counts 1 and 3 do not raise the hips or arch the back to assume the vertical position.

Precautions: Soldiers should not jerk on the head or neck to assume the vertical position.

Conditioning Drill 2
Exercise 3: The Pull-up

Purpose: This exercise strengthens the forearm, arm and back muscles.

Starting Position: Extended hang using the overhand grip with the thumbs around the bar.

Cadence: MODERATE.

Count:
1. Pull the body upward keeping the body straight until the chin is above the bar.
2. Return to the Starting Position in a controlled manner.

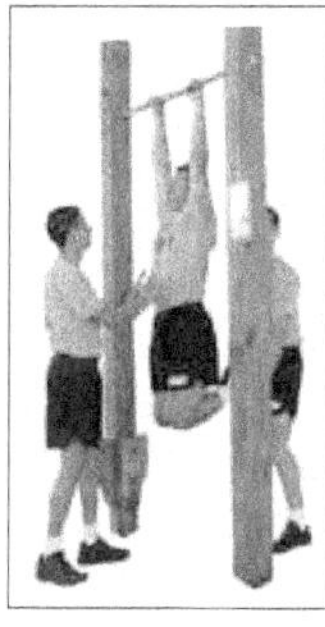

Starting Position

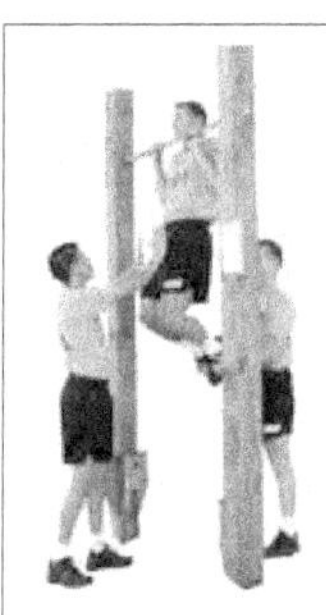

Count 1

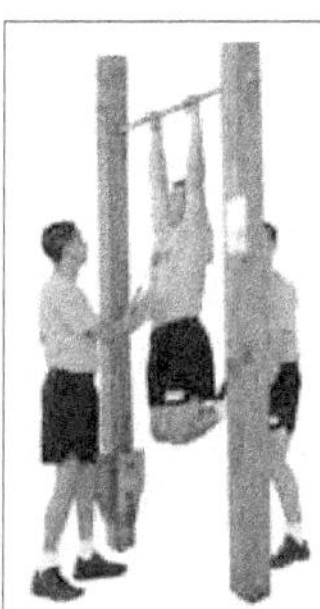

Count 2

Hand Positions:

The hand position is for the pull-up is the overhand grip, with the palms facing away from the face.

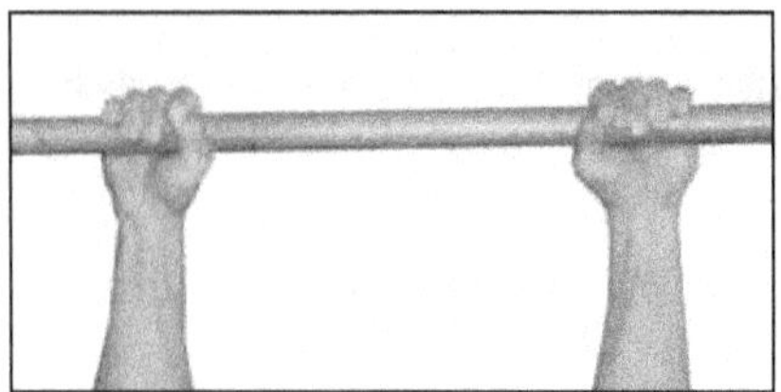

Check Points:

- ❑ Throughout the exercise keep the feet and legs together.
- ❑ Throughout the exercise, arms are shoulder width, palms facing away from the body, with thumbs around the bar.
- ❑ Avoid kicking or swinging to achieve the up position.

Precautions: Spotters standing to the front and rear of the exerciser are used to ensure precision and safety by assisting Soldiers when fatigued or unable to properly execute the desired number of repetitions. As Soldiers become more proficient, they will need less assistance and will eventually be able to perform the exercises unassisted. Spotters must provide as much or as little assistance as needed so that the exercise is performed with precision.

Conditioning Drill 3
Exercise 1: The Power Jump

Purpose: This exercise reinforces correct jumping and landing, stimulates balance and coordination, and develops explosive strength.

Starting Position: Straddle stance with hands on hips.

Cadence: MODERATE.

Count:
1. Squat with the heels flat as the spine rounds forward to allow the straight arms to reach to the ground, touching with the palms of the hands.
2. Jump forcefully into the air, vigorously raising arms overhead, with palms facing inward.
3. Control the landing and repeat Count 1.
4. Return to the Starting Position.

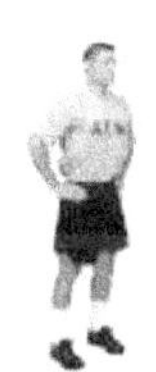

Starting Position

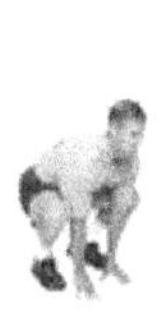

Count 1

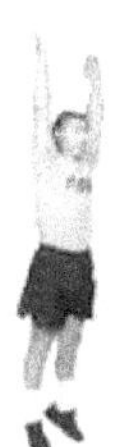

Count 2

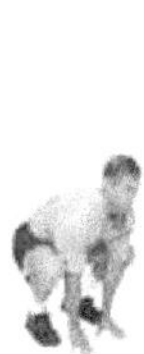

Count 3

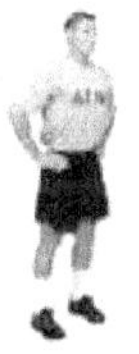

Starting Position

Check Points:

- At the Starting Position, tighten the abdominals to stabilize the trunk.
- On Counts 1 and 3, keep the back generally straight with the head up and eyes forward.
- On Count 2 the arms should be extended fully overhead. The trunk and legs should also be in line.
- On each landing, the feet should be directed forward and maintained at shoulder distance apart. The landing should be "soft" and proceed from balls of the feet to the heels. The vertical line from the shoulders through the knees to the balls of the feet should be demonstrated on each landing.

Precautions: N/A.

Conditioning Drill 3
Exercise 2: The V-up

Purpose: This exercise develops the abdominal and hip flexor muscles while enhancing balance.

Starting Position: Supine, arms on ground 45-degrees to the side, palms down with fingers spread. The chin is tucked and the head is 1-2 inches off the ground.

Cadence: MODERATE.

Count:
1. Raise straight legs and trunk to form a V-position, using arms as needed.
2. Return to the Starting Position.
3. Repeat Count 1.
4. Return to the Starting Position.

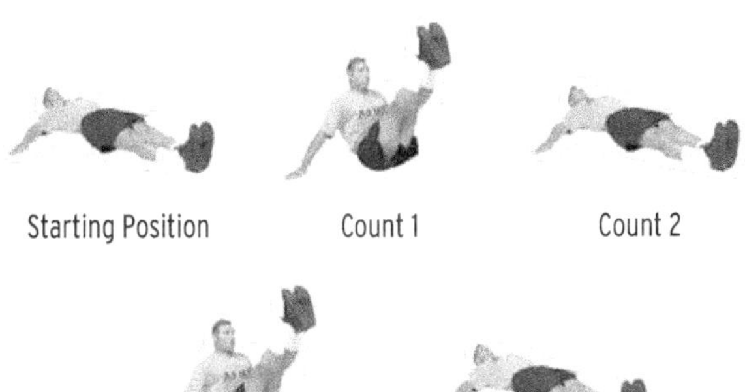

Starting Position | Count 1 | Count 2

Count 3 | Starting Position

Check Points:

- ❑ At the Starting Position, tighten the abdominal muscles to tilt the pelvis and the lower back toward the ground.
- ❑ On Counts 1 and 3, the knees and trunk are straight with the head in line with the trunk.

Precautions: To protect the spine, do not jerk the legs and trunk to rise to the V-position.

Conditioning Drill 3
Exercise 3: The Mountain Climber

Purpose: This exercise develops the ability to quickly move the legs to power out of the front leaning rest position.

Starting Position: Front leaning rest position with the left foot below the chest and between the arms.

Cadence: MODERATE.

Count:
1. Push upward with the feet and quickly change positions of the legs.
2. Return to the Starting Position.
3. Repeat the movements in Count 1.
4. Return to the Starting Position.

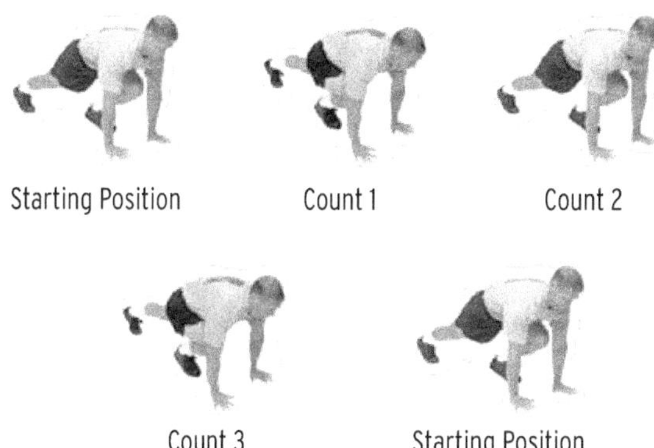

Starting Position   Count 1   Count 2

Count 3   Starting Position

Check Points:

- ❏ The hands are directly below the shoulders with fingers spread (middle fingers point straight ahead) with the elbows straight, not locked.
- ❏ The trunk must not sag. To prevent, tighten the abdominal muscles and maintain this contraction throughout the exercise.
- ❏ The head is aligned with the spine and the eyes are directed to a point approximately two feet in front of the body.
- ❏ Throughout the exercise, remain on the balls of the feet.
- ❏ Move the legs straight forward and backward, not at angles.

Precautions: N/A.

Conditioning Drill 3
Exercise 4: The Leg Tuck and Twist

Purpose: This exercise develops trunk strength and mobility while enhancing balance.

Starting Position: Seated with trunk straight but leaning backward 45-degrees, arms straight, and hands on ground 45-degrees to the rear, palms down, with fingers spread. Legs are straight, extended to the front and 8-12 inches off the ground.

Cadence: MODERATE.

Count:

1. Raise legs while rotating on to the left buttock and draw the knees toward the left shoulder.
2. Return to the Starting Position.
3. Repeat Count 1 in the opposite direction.
4. Return to the Starting Position.

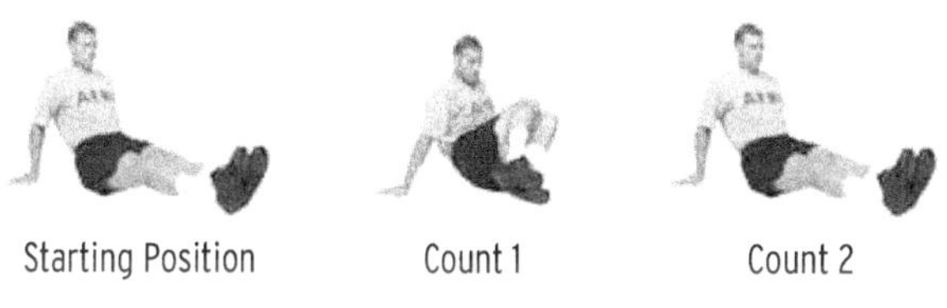

Starting Position   Count 1   Count 2

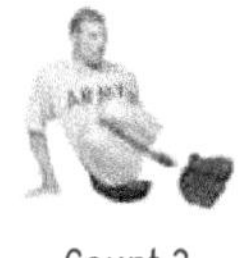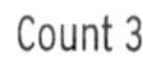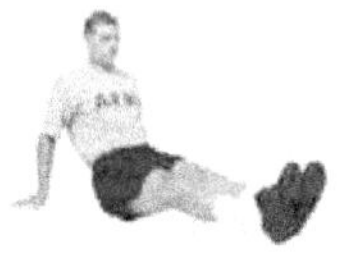

Count 3   Starting Position

Check Points:

❏ At the Starting Position, tighten the abdominals to stabilize the trunk.
❏ On all counts, the legs and knees stay together.
❏ On Counts 1 and 3, the head and trunk remain still as the legs move.
❏ On Counts 1 and 3, the legs are tucked (bent) and aligned diagonal to the trunk.

Precautions: To protect the back on Counts 1 and 3, do not jerk the legs and trunk to achieve the end position.

Conditioning Drill 3
Exercise 5: The Single-leg Push-up

Purpose: This exercise strengthens muscles of the chest, shoulders, arms, and trunk. Raising one leg while maintaining proper trunk position makes this an excellent trunk stabilizing exercise.

Starting Position: Front-leaning rest position.

Cadence: MODERATE.

Count:
1. Bend the elbows, lowering the body until the upper arms are parallel with the ground while raising the left leg until 8-10 inches off the ground.
2. Return to the Starting Position.
3. Repeat Count 1, bringing the right leg to 8-10 inches off the ground.
4. Return to the Starting Position.

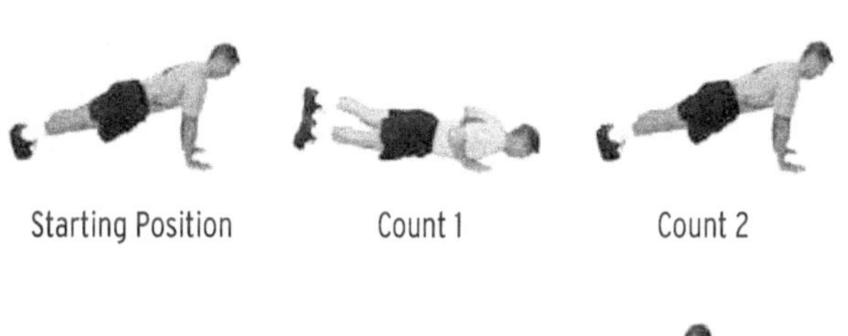

Starting Position	Count 1	Count 2

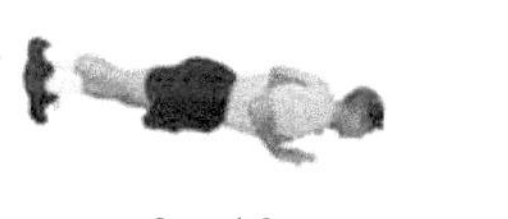
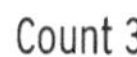
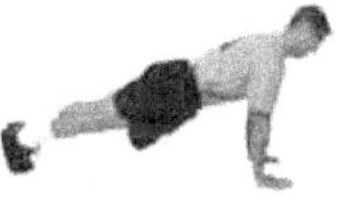

Count 3	Starting Position

Check Points:

❑ Perform a squat thrust to move into the front leaning rest, maintaining the body straight from head to heels. Body weight is supported on the hands and balls of the feet.

❑ The fingers should be extended and spread so the middle fingers point straight ahead and are directly in line with the shoulders.

❑ On Counts 1 and 3, the upper arms stay close to the trunk.

❑ On Counts 2 and 4, the elbows straighten but do not lock.

❑ On Counts 1 and 3, the raised leg is straight and aligned with the trunk.

❑ The trunk must not sag. To prevent this, tighten the abdominal muscles while in the Starting Position and maintain this contraction throughout the exercise.

Precautions: Do not jerk the leg to be raised past straight alignment with the trunk, as this may place undue stress on the back.

TRAINING SCHEDULES

The four training schedules below are tailored based on your performance of the 1-1-1 Physical Fitness Assessment. Use the one that is appropriate to your individual needs.

- **Training schedule #1** is the training schedule for the Future Soldier who passes all the events on the initial 1-1-1 Physical Fitness Assessment.

- **Training schedule #2** is the training schedule for the Future Soldier who passes the push-ups and sit-ups but fails the one-mile run on the initial 1-1-1 Physical Fitness Assessment.

- **Training schedule #3** is the training schedule for the Future Soldier who fails the push-ups and/or sit-ups but passes the one-mile run on the initial 1-1-1 Physical Fitness Assessment.

- **Training schedule #4** is the training schedule for the Future Soldier who fails the push-ups and/or sit-ups and the one-mile run on the initial 1-1-1 Physical Fitness Assessment.

- **Blank training schedules** are included for you to track your own training program.

- **Personal Training Assessment** forms are included for you to track your progress on the 1-1-1 Physical Fitness Assessment exercises.

USING THE TRAINING SCHEDULES

WARM-UP	CD1 & MMD		
ACTIVITY	Run 20 minutes		
	Male A	B	C
	7:15	8:00	8:45
	Female A	B	C
	9:15	10:00	11:00
COOL-DOWN	SD		

WARM-UP	4C, HSD & CD1
ACTIVITY	CD2 15/15/5 repetitions
	CD3 5 repetitions
COOL-DOWN	SD

This means perform 5 repetitions of each exercise in Conditioning Drill 1 (CD1) and 1 repetition of each exercise in The Military Movement Drill (MMD).

This means run for 20 minutes at the pace listed for your ability group. For example: A male in group A should run 20 minutes at a 7:15 per mile pace (almost 3 miles total).

This means perform 4 for the Core, The Hip Stability Drill, and 5 repetitions of Conditioning Drill 1 (CD1).

This means perform 15 repetitions of the push-up and sit-up, and 5 pull-ups in Conditioning Drill 2 (CD2). (Push-ups and sit-ups are 4-count exercises.)

This means perform 5 repetitions of each exercise in Conditioning Drill 3 (CD3).

This means perform the stretch drill holding each stretch for 20 seconds.

TRAINING SCHEDULE 1

		SUNDAY	MONDAY	TUESDAY	WEDNESDAY
WEEK ONE	WARM-UP	REST	CD1 & MMD	4C, HSD & CD1	CD1 & MMD
	ACTIVITY		Run 15 minutes	CD2 (10/10/5 reps x 1 set)	30:60s (6 reps)
			Male A B C	CD3 (5 reps x 1 set)	
			7:30 8:15 9:00		
			Female A B C		
			9:30 10:15 11:15		
	COOL-DOWN		SD	SD	SD
WEEK TWO	WARM-UP	REST	CD1 & MMD	4C, HSD & CD1	CD1 & MMD
	ACTIVITY		Run 20 minutes	CD2 (10/10/5 reps x 1 set)	30:60s (6 reps)
			Male A B C	CD3 (5 reps x 1 set)	
			7:30 8:15 9:00		
			Female A B C		
			9:30 10:15 11:15		
	COOL-DOWN		SD	SD	SD
WEEK THREE	WARM-UP	REST	CD1 & MMD	4C, HSD & CD1	CD1 & MMD
	ACTIVITY		Run 20 minutes	CD2 (10/10/5 reps x 2 sets)	30:60s (7 reps)
			Male A B C	CD3 (5 reps x 1 set)	
			7:30 8:15 9:00		
			Female A B C		
			9:30 10:15 11:15		
	COOL-DOWN		SD	SD	SD
WEEK FOUR	WARM-UP	REST	CD1 & MMD	4C, HSD & CD1	CD1 & MMD
	ACTIVITY		Run 20 minutes	CD2 (10/10/5 reps x 2 sets)	30:60s (7 reps)
			Male A B C	CD3 (5 reps x 1 set)	
			7:30 8:15 9:00		
			Female A B C		
			9:30 10:15 11:15		
	COOL-DOWN		SD	SD	SD

TRAINING SCHEDULE 1
(continued)

			THURSDAY	FRIDAY	SATURDAY
WEEK ONE	WARM-UP		4C, HSD & CD1	CD1 & MMD	REST
	ACTIVITY		CD2 (10/10/5 reps x 1 set)	Run 15 minutes	
			CD3 (5 reps x 1 set)	Male A B C	
				7:30 8:15 9:00	
				Female A B C	
				9:30 10:15 11:15	
	COOL-DOWN		SD	SD	
WEEK TWO	WARM-UP		4C, HSD & CD1	CD1 & MMD	REST
	ACTIVITY		CD2 (10/10/5 reps x 1 set)	Run 20 minutes	
			CD3 (5 reps x 1 set)	Male A B C	
				7:30 8:15 9:00	
				Female A B C	
				9:30 10:15 11:15	
	COOL-DOWN		SD	SD	
WEEK THREE	WARM-UP		4C, HSD & CD1	CD1 & MMD	REST
	ACTIVITY		CD2 (10/10/5 reps x 2 sets)	Run 20 minutes	
			CD3 (5 reps x 1 set)	Male A B C	
				7:30 8:15 9:00	
				Female A B C	
				9:30 10:15 11:15	
	COOL-DOWN		SD	SD	
WEEK FOUR	WARM-UP		4C, HSD & CD1	REST	1-1-1 PHYSICAL FITNESS ASSESSMENT
	ACTIVITY		CD2 (10/10/5 reps x 2 sets)		
			CD3 (5 reps x 1 set)		
	COOL-DOWN		SD		

YEAR

MONTH

TRAINING SCHEDULE 1
(continued)

			SUNDAY	MONDAY	TUESDAY	WEDNESDAY
WEEK FIVE		WARM-UP	REST	CD1 & MMD	4C, HSD & CD1	CD1 & MMD
		ACTIVITY		Run 20 minutes	CD2 (15/15/5 reps x 1 set)	30:60s (8 reps)
				Male A B C	CD3 (5 reps x 1 set)	
				7:15 8:00 8:45		
				Female A B C		
				9:15 10:00 11:00		
		COOL-DOWN		SD	SD	SD
WEEK SIX		WARM-UP	REST	CD1 & MMD	4C, HSD & CD1	CD1 & MMD
		ACTIVITY		Run 20 minutes	CD2 (15/15/5 reps x 1 set)	30:60s (8 reps)
				Male A B C	CD3 (5 reps x 1 set)	
				7:15 8:00 8:45		
				Female A B C		
				9:15 10:00 11:00		
		COOL-DOWN		SD	SD	SD
WEEK SEVEN		WARM-UP	REST	CD1 & MMD	4C, HSD & CD1	CD1 & MMD
		ACTIVITY		Run 20 minutes	CD2 (15/15/5 reps x 1 set)	30:60s (9 reps)
				Male A B C	CD3 (10 reps x 1 set)	
				7:15 8:00 8:45		
				Female A B C		
				9:15 10:00 11:00		
		COOL-DOWN		SD	SD	SD
WEEK EIGHT		WARM-UP	REST	CD1 & MMD	4C, HSD & CD1	CD1 & MMD
		ACTIVITY		Run 20 minutes	CD2 (15/15/5 reps x 1 set)	30:60s (9 reps)
				Male A B C	CD3 (10 reps x 1 set)	
				7:15 8:00 8:45		
				Female A B C		
				9:15 10:00 11:00		
		COOL-DOWN		SD	SD	SD

TRAINING SCHEDULE 1
(continued)

		THURSDAY	FRIDAY	SATURDAY	
WEEK FIVE	WARM-UP	4C, HSD & CD1	CD1 & MMD	REST	
	ACTIVITY	CD2 (15/15/5 reps x 1 set)	Run 20 minutes		
		CD3 (5 reps x 1 set)	Male A B C		
			7:15 8:00 8:45		
			Female A B C		
			9:15 10:00 11:00		
	COOL-DOWN	SD	SD		
WEEK SIX	WARM-UP	4C, HSD & CD1	CD1 & MMD	REST	
	ACTIVITY	CD2 (15/15/5 reps x 1 set)	Run 20 minutes		
		CD3 (5 reps x 1 set)	Male A B C		
			7:15 8:00 8:45		
			Female A B C		
			9:15 10:00 11:00		
	COOL-DOWN	SD	SD		
WEEK SEVEN	WARM-UP	4C, HSD & CD1	CD1 & MMD	REST	
	ACTIVITY	CD2 (15/15/5 reps x 1 set)	Run 20 minutes		
		CD3 (10 reps x 1 set)	Male A B C		
			7:15 8:00 8:45		
			Female A B C		
			9:15 10:00 11:00		
	COOL-DOWN	SD	SD		
WEEK EIGHT	WARM-UP	4C, HSD & CD1			
	ACTIVITY	CD2 (15/15/5 reps x 1 set)			
		CD3 (10 reps x 1 set)	REST	1-1-1 PHYSICAL FITNESS ASSESSMENT	
	COOL-DOWN	SD			

YEAR

MONTH

TRAINING SCHEDULE 1
(continued)

			SUNDAY	MONDAY	TUESDAY	WEDNESDAY
WEEK NINE		WARM-UP	REST	CD1 & MMD	4C, HSD & CD1	CD1 & MMD
		ACTIVITY		Run 20 minutes	CD2 (15/15/5 reps x 2 sets)	30:60s (10 reps)
				Male A B C	CD3 (10 reps x 1 set)	
				7:00 7:45 8:30		
				Female A B C		
				9:00 9:45 10:45		
		COOL-DOWN		SD	SD	SD
WEEK TEN		WARM-UP	REST	CD1 & MMD	4C, HSD & CD1	CD1 & MMD
		ACTIVITY		Run 20 minutes	CD2 (15/15/5 reps x 2 sets)	30:60s (10 reps)
				Male A B C	CD3 (10 reps x 1 set)	
				7:00 7:45 8:30		
				Female A B C		
				9:00 9:45 10:45		
		COOL-DOWN		SD	SD	SD
WEEK ELEVEN		WARM-UP	REST	CD1 & MMD	4C, HSD & CD1	CD1 & MMD
		ACTIVITY		Run 20 minutes	CD2 (20/20/5 reps x 1 set)	30:60s (10 reps)
				Male A B C	CD3 (10 reps x 1 set)	
				7:00 7:30 8:15		
				Female A B C		
				9:00 9:30 10:30		
		COOL-DOWN		SD	SD	SD
WEEK TWELVE		WARM-UP	REST	CD1 & MMD	4C, HSD & CD1	CD1 & MMD
		ACTIVITY		Run 20 minutes	CD2 (20/20/5 reps x 1 set)	30:60s (10 reps)
				Male A B C	CD3 (10 reps x 1 set)	
				7:00 7:30 8:15		
				Female A B C		
				9:00 9:30 10:30		
		COOL-DOWN		SD	SD	SD

TRAINING SCHEDULE 1
(continued)

		THURSDAY	FRIDAY	SATURDAY
WEEK NINE	WARM-UP	4C, HSD & CD1	CD1 & MMD	REST
	ACTIVITY	CD2 (15/15/5 reps x 2 sets)	Run 20 minutes	
		CD3 (10 reps x 1 set)	Male A B C	
			7:00 7:45 8:30	
			Female A B C	
			9:00 9:45 10:45	
	COOL-DOWN	SD	SD	
WEEK TEN	WARM-UP	4C, HSD & CD1	CD1 & MMD	REST
	ACTIVITY	CD2 (15/15/5 reps x 2 sets)	Run 20 minutes	
		CD3 (10 reps x 1 set)	Male A B C	
			7:00 7:45 8:30	
			Female A B C	
			9:00 9:45 10:45	
	COOL-DOWN	SD	SD	
WEEK ELEVEN	WARM-UP	4C, HSD & CD1	CD1 & MMD	REST
	ACTIVITY	CD2 (20/20/5 reps x 1 set)	Run 20 minutes	
		CD3 (10 reps x 1 set)	Male A B C	
			7:00 7:30 8:15	
			Female A B C	
			9:00 9:30 10:30	
	COOL-DOWN	SD	SD	
WEEK TWELVE	WARM-UP	4C, HSD & CD1	REST	1-1-1 PHYSICAL FITNESS ASSESSMENT
	ACTIVITY	CD2 (20/20/5 reps x 1 set)		
		CD3 (10 reps x 1 set)		
	COOL-DOWN	SD		

YEAR

MONTH

TRAINING SCHEDULE 1
Maintenance Phase

	MONDAY	TUESDAY	WEDNESDAY	THURSDAY	FRIDAY
WARM-UP	CD1 & MMD	4C, HSD & CD1	CD1 & MMD	4C, HSD & CD1	CD1 & MMD
ACTIVITY	A & B Run 30 minutes	CD2 (20/20/5 reps x 1 set)	30:60s (10 reps)	CD2 (20/20/5 reps x 1 set)	A & B Run 30 minutes
	C Run 20 minutes	CD3 (10 reps x 1 set)		CD3 (10 reps x 1 set)	C Run 20 minutes
	A B C				A B C
	7:30 8:00 9:30				7:30 8:00 9:30
COOL-DOWN	SD	SD	SD	SD	SD

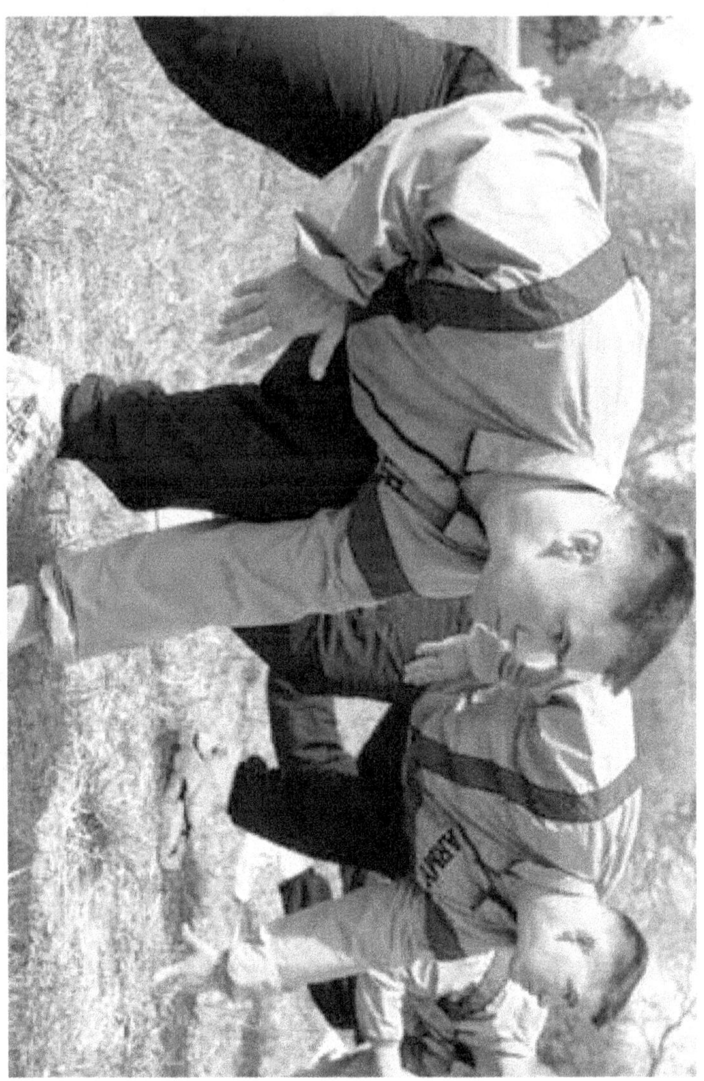

TRAINING SCHEDULE 2

		SUNDAY	MONDAY	TUESDAY	WEDNESDAY
WEEK ONE	WARM-UP	REST	CD1 & MMD	4C, HSD & CD1	CD1 & MMD
	ACTIVITY		Walk 4 min. Run 2 min. (5x)	CD2 (10/10/5 reps x 1 set)	30:60s (4 reps)
				CD3 (5 reps x 1 set)	
	COOL-DOWN		SD	SD	SD
WEEK TWO	WARM-UP	REST	CD1 & MMD	4C, HSD & CD1	CD1 & MMD
	ACTIVITY		Walk 3 min. Run 3 min. (5x)	CD2 (10/10/5 reps x 1 set)	30:60s (4 reps)
				CD3 (5 reps x 1 set)	
	COOL-DOWN		SD	SD	SD
WEEK THREE	WARM-UP	REST	CD1 & MMD	4C, HSD & CD1	CD1 & MMD
	ACTIVITY		Walk 2 min. Run 4 min. (5x)	CD2 (10/10/5 reps x 2 sets)	30:60s (5 reps)
				CD3 (5 reps x 1 set)	
	COOL-DOWN		SD	SD	SD
WEEK FOUR	WARM-UP	REST	CD1 & MMD	4C, HSD & CD1	CD1 & MMD
	ACTIVITY		Walk 2 min. Run 4 min. (5x)	CD2 (10/10/5 reps x 2 sets)	30:60s (5 reps)
				CD3 (5 reps x 1 set)	
	COOL-DOWN		SD	SD	SD

TRAINING SCHEDULE 2
(continued)

		THURSDAY	FRIDAY	SATURDAY	
WEEK ONE	WARM-UP	4C, HSD & CD1	CD1 & MMD	REST	
	ACTIVITY	CD2 (10/10/5 reps x 1 set)	Walk 4 min. Run 2 min. (5x)		
		CD3 (5 reps x 1 set)			
	COOL-DOWN	SD	SD		
WEEK TWO	WARM-UP	4C, HSD & CD1	CD1 & MMD	REST	
	ACTIVITY	CD2 (10/10/5 reps x 1 set)	Walk 3 min. Run 3 min. (5x)		
		CD3 (5 reps x 1 set)			
	COOL-DOWN	SD	SD		
WEEK THREE	WARM-UP	4C, HSD & CD1	CD1 & MMD	REST	
	ACTIVITY	CD2 (10/10/5 reps x 2 sets)	Walk 2 min. Run 4 min. (5x)		
		CD3 (5 reps x 1 set)			
	COOL-DOWN	SD	SD		
WEEK FOUR	WARM-UP	4C, HSD & CD1	REST	1-1-1 PHYSICAL FITNESS ASSESSMENT	
	ACTIVITY	CD2 (10/10/5 reps x 2 sets)			
		CD3 (5 reps x 1 set)			
	COOL-DOWN	SD			

YEAR

MONTH

TRAINING SCHEDULE 2
(continued)

		SUNDAY	MONDAY	TUESDAY	WEDNESDAY
WEEK FIVE	WARM-UP	REST	CD1 & MMD	4C, HSD & CD1	CD1 & MMD
	ACTIVITY		Run 10 minutes	CD2 (15/15/5 reps x 1 set)	30:60s (6 reps)
				CD3 (5 reps x 1 set)	
	COOL-DOWN		SD	SD	SD
WEEK SIX	WARM-UP	REST	CD1 & MMD	4C, HSD & CD1	CD1 & MMD
	ACTIVITY		Run 12 minutes	CD2 (15/15/5 reps x 1 set)	30:60s (6 reps)
				CD3 (5 reps x 1 set)	
	COOL-DOWN		SD	SD	SD
WEEK SEVEN	WARM-UP	REST	CD1 & MMD	4C, HSD & CD1	CD1 & MMD
	ACTIVITY		Run 1 mile	CD2 (15/15/5 reps x 1 set)	30:60s (7 reps)
			M: 9:30/F: 11:30	CD3 (10 reps x 1 set)	
	COOL-DOWN		SD	SD	SD
WEEK EIGHT	WARM-UP	REST	CD1 & MMD	4C, HSD & CD1	CD1 & MMD
	ACTIVITY		Run 1 mile	CD2 (15/15/5 reps x 1 set)	30:60s (7 reps)
			M: 9:15/F: 11:15	CD3 (10 reps x 1 set)	
	COOL-DOWN		SD	SD	SD

TRAINING SCHEDULE 2
(continued)

		THURSDAY	FRIDAY	SATURDAY	
WEEK FIVE	WARM-UP	4C, HSD & CD1	CD1 & MMD	REST	
	ACTIVITY	CD2 (15/15/5 reps x 1 set)	Run 10 minutes		
		CD3 (5 reps x 1 set)			
	COOL-DOWN	SD	SD		
WEEK SIX	WARM-UP	4C, HSD & CD1	CD1 & MMD	REST	
	ACTIVITY	CD2 (15/15/5 reps x 1 set)	Run 12 minutes		
		CD3 (5 reps x 1 set)			
	COOL-DOWN	SD	SD		
WEEK SEVEN	WARM-UP	4C, HSD & CD1	CD1 & MMD	REST	
	ACTIVITY	CD2 (15/15/5 reps x 1 set)	Run 1 mile		
		CD3 (10 reps x 1 set)	M: 9:30/F: 11:30		
	COOL-DOWN	SD	SD		
WEEK EIGHT	WARM-UP	4C, HSD & CD1	REST	1-1-1 PHYSICAL FITNESS ASSESSMENT	
	ACTIVITY	CD2 (15/15/5 reps x 1 set)			
		CD3 (10 reps x 1 set)			
	COOL-DOWN	SD			

YEAR

MONTH

TRAINING SCHEDULE 2
(continued)

		SUNDAY	MONDAY	TUESDAY	WEDNESDAY
WEEK NINE	WARM-UP	REST	CD1 & MMD	4C, HSD & CD1	CD1 & MMD
	ACTIVITY		Run 1 mile	CD2 (15/15/5 reps x 2 sets)	30:60s (8 reps)
			M: 9:00/F: 11:00	CD3 (10 reps x 1 set)	
	COOL-DOWN		SD	SD	SD
WEEK TEN	WARM-UP	REST	CD1 & MMD	4C, HSD & CD1	CD1 & MMD
	ACTIVITY		Run 1 mile	CD2 (15/15/5 reps x 2 sets)	30:60s (8 reps)
			M: 8:45/F: 10:45	CD3 (10 reps x 1 set)	
	COOL-DOWN		SD	SD	SD
WEEK ELEVEN	WARM-UP	REST	CD1 & MMD	4C, HSD & CD1	CD1 & MMD
	ACTIVITY		Run 1 mile	CD2 (20/20/5 reps x 1 set)	30:60s (8 reps)
			M: 8:30/F: 10:30	CD3 (10 reps x 1 set)	
	COOL-DOWN		SD	SD	SD
WEEK TWELVE	WARM-UP	REST	CD1 & MMD	4C, HSD & CD1	CD1 & MMD
	ACTIVITY		Run 1 mile	CD2 (20/20/5 reps x 1 set)	30:60s (8 reps)
			M: 8:15/F: 10:15	CD3 (10 reps x 1 set)	
	COOL-DOWN		SD	SD	SD

TRAINING SCHEDULE 2
(continued)

		WEEK TWELVE	WEEK ELEVEN	WEEK TEN	WEEK NINE
THURSDAY	WARM-UP	4C, HSD & CD1	4C, HSD & CD1	4C, HSD & CD1	4C, HSD & CD1
	ACTIVITY	CD2 (20/20/5 reps x 1 set); CD3 (10 reps x 1 set)	CD2 (20/20/5 reps x 1 set); CD3 (10 reps x 1 set)	CD2 (15/15/5 reps x 2 sets); CD3 (10 reps x 1 set)	CD2 (15/15/5 reps x 2 sets); CD3 (10 reps x 1 set)
	COOL-DOWN	SD	SD	SD	SD
FRIDAY	WARM-UP	REST	CD1 & MMD	CD1 & MMD	CD1 & MMD
	ACTIVITY		Run 1 mile	Run 1 mile	Run 1 mile
	COOL-DOWN		M: 8:30/F: 10:30; SD	M: 8:45/F: 10:45; SD	M: 9:00/F: 11:00; SD
SATURDAY		1-1-1 PHYSICAL FITNESS ASSESSMENT	REST	REST	REST

MONTH   YEAR

TRAINING SCHEDULE 2
Maintenance Phase

	MONDAY	TUESDAY	WEDNESDAY	THURSDAY	FRIDAY
WARM-UP	CD1 & MMD	4C, HSD & CD1	CD1 & MMD	4C, HSD & CD1	CD1 & MMD
ACTIVITY	Run 20-30 minutes	CD2 (20/20/5 reps x 1 set)	30:60s (10 reps)	CD2 (20/20/5 reps x 1 set)	Run 20-30 minutes
		CD3 (10 reps x 1 set)		CD3 (10 reps x 1 set)	
COOL-DOWN	SD	SD	SD	SD	SD

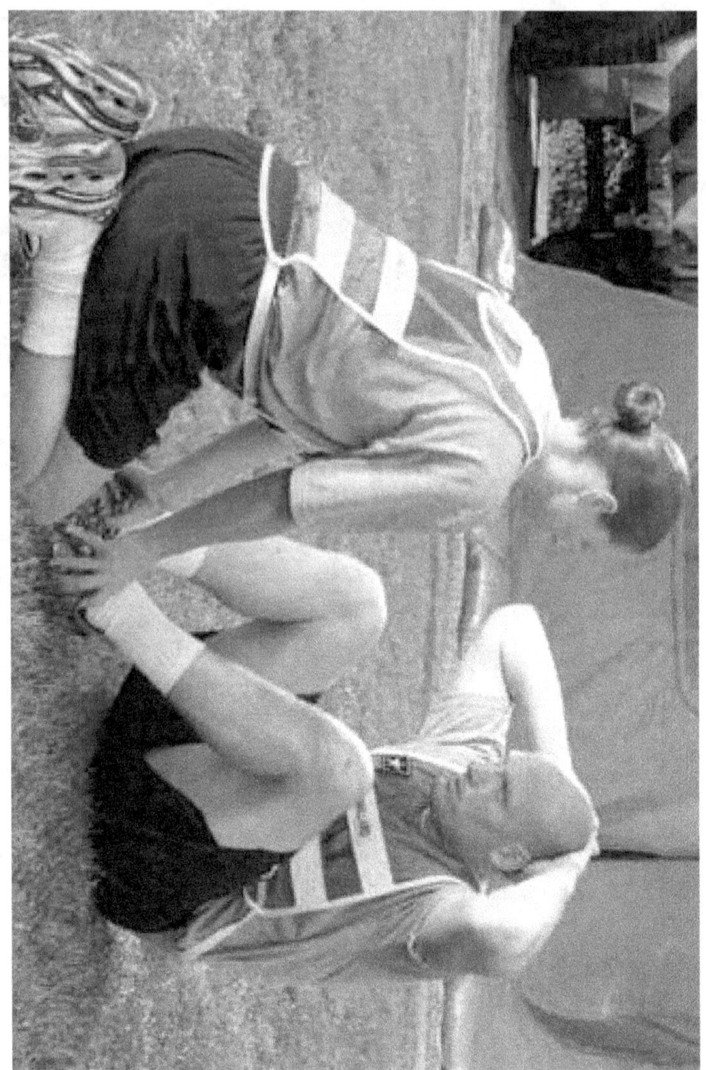

TRAINING SCHEDULE 3

			SUNDAY	MONDAY	TUESDAY	WEDNESDAY
WEEK ONE		WARM-UP	REST	CD1 & MMD	4C, HSD & CD1	CD1 & MMD
		ACTIVITY		Run 15 minutes	CD2 (5/5/2 reps x 2 sets)	30:60s (6 reps)
				Male A B C		
				7:30 8:15 9:00		
				Female A B C		
				9:30 10:15 11:15		
		COOL-DOWN		SD	SD	SD
WEEK TWO		WARM-UP	REST	CD1 & MMD	4C, HSD & CD1	CD1 & MMD
		ACTIVITY		Run 20 minutes	CD2 (6/6/3 reps x 2 sets)	30:60s (6 reps)
				Male A B C		
				7:30 8:15 9:00		
				Female A B C		
				9:30 10:15 11:15		
		COOL-DOWN		SD	SD	SD
WEEK THREE		WARM-UP	REST	CD1 & MMD	4C, HSD & CD1	CD1 & MMD
		ACTIVITY		Run 20 minutes	CD2 7/7/4 reps x 2 sets)	30:60s (7 reps)
				Male A B C		
				7:30 8:15 9:00		
				Female A B C		
				9:30 10:15 11:15		
		COOL-DOWN		SD	SD	SD
WEEK FOUR		WARM-UP	REST	CD1 & MMD	4C, HSD & CD1	CD1 & MMD
		ACTIVITY		Run 20 minutes	CD2 (8/8/4 reps x 2 sets)	30:60s (7 reps)
				Male A B C		
				7:30 8:15 9:00		
				Female A B C		
				9:30 10:15 11:15		
		COOL-DOWN		SD	SD	SD

TRAINING SCHEDULE 3
(continued)

			THURSDAY	FRIDAY	SATURDAY	
WEEK ONE		WARM-UP	4C, HSD & CD1	CD1 & MMD	REST	**YEAR**
		ACTIVITY	CD2 (5/5/2 reps x 2 sets)	Run 15 minutes		
				Male A B C		
				7:30 8:15 9:00		
				Female A B C		
				9:30 10:15 11:15		
		COOL-DOWN	SD	SD		
WEEK TWO		WARM-UP	4C, HSD & CD1	CD1 & MMD	REST	
		ACTIVITY	CD2 (6/6/3 reps x 2 sets)	Run 20 minutes		
				Male A B C		
				7:30 8:15 9:00		
				Female A B C		
				9:30 10:15 11:15		
		COOL-DOWN	SD	SD		
WEEK THREE		WARM-UP	4C, HSD & CD1	CD1 & MMD	REST	
		ACTIVITY	CD2 7/7/4 reps x 2 sets	Run 20 minutes		
				Male A B C		
				7:30 8:15 9:00		
				Female A B C		
				9:30 10:15 11:15		**MONTH**
		COOL-DOWN	SD	SD		
WEEK FOUR		WARM-UP	4C, HSD & CD1			
		ACTIVITY	CD2 (8/8/4 reps x 2 sets)			
				REST	1-1-1 PHYSICAL FITNESS ASSESSMENT	
		COOL-DOWN	SD			

TRAINING SCHEDULE 3
(continued)

			SUNDAY	MONDAY	TUESDAY	WEDNESDAY
WEEK FIVE		WARM-UP	REST	CD1 & MMD	4C, HSD & CD1	CD1 & MMD
		ACTIVITY		Run 20 minutes	CD2 (10/10/5 reps x 1 set)	30:60s (8 reps)
				Male A B C	CD3 (5 reps x 1 set)	
				7:15 8:00 8:45		
				Female A B C		
				9:15 10:00 11:00		
		COOL-DOWN		SD	SD	SD
WEEK SIX		WARM-UP	REST	CD1 & MMD	4C, HSD & CD1	CD1 & MMD
		ACTIVITY		Run 20 minutes	CD2 (10/10/5 reps x 1 set)	30:60s (8 reps)
				Male A B C	CD3 (5 reps x 1 set)	
				7:15 8:00 8:45		
				Female A B C		
				9:15 10:00 11:00		
		COOL-DOWN		SD	SD	SD
WEEK SEVEN		WARM-UP	REST	CD1 & MMD	4C, HSD & CD1	CD1 & MMD
		ACTIVITY		Run 20 minutes	CD2 (10/10/5 reps x 1 set)	30:60s (9 reps)
				Male A B C	CD3 (5 reps x 1 set)	
				7:15 8:00 8:45		
				Female A B C		
				9:15 10:00 11:00		
		COOL-DOWN		SD	SD	SD
WEEK EIGHT		WARM-UP	REST	CD1 & MMD	4C, HSD & CD1	CD1 & MMD
		ACTIVITY		Run 20 minutes	CD2 (10/10/5 reps x 1 set)	30:60s (9 reps)
				Male A B C	CD3 (5 reps x 1 set)	
				7:15 8:00 8:45		
				Female A B C		
				9:15 10:00 11:00		
		COOL-DOWN		SD	SD	SD

TRAINING SCHEDULE 3
(continued)

			THURSDAY	FRIDAY	SATURDAY	
WEEK FIVE	WARM-UP		4C, HSD & CD1	CD1 & MMD	REST	YEAR
	ACTIVITY		CD2 (10/10/5 reps x 1 set)	Run 20 minutes		
			CD3 (5 reps x 1 set)	Male A B C		
				7:15 8:00 8:45		
				Female A B C		
				9:15 10:00 11:00		
	COOL-DOWN		SD	SD		
WEEK SIX	WARM-UP		4C, HSD & CD1	CD1 & MMD	REST	
	ACTIVITY		CD2 (10/10/5 reps x 1 set)	Run 20 minutes		
			CD3 (5 reps x 1 set)	Male A B C		
				7:15 8:00 8:45		
				Female A B C		
				9:15 10:00 11:00		
	COOL-DOWN		SD	SD		
WEEK SEVEN	WARM-UP		4C, HSD & CD1	CD1 & MMD	REST	MONTH
	ACTIVITY		CD2 (10/10/5 reps x 1 set)	Run 20 minutes		
			CD3 (5 reps x 1 set)	Male A B C		
				7:15 8:00 8:45		
				Female A B C		
				9:15 10:00 11:00		
	COOL-DOWN		SD	SD		
WEEK EIGHT	WARM-UP		4C, HSD & CD1	REST	1-1-1 PHYSICAL FITNESS ASSESSMENT	
	ACTIVITY		CD2 (10/10/5 reps x 1 set)			
			CD3 (5 reps x 1 set)			
	COOL-DOWN		SD			

TRAINING SCHEDULE 3
(continued)

Day		WEEK NINE	WEEK TEN	WEEK ELEVEN	WEEK TWELVE
SUNDAY		REST	REST	REST	REST
MONDAY	WARM-UP	CD1 & MMD	CD1 & MMD	CD1 & MMD	CD1 & MMD
	ACTIVITY	Run 20 minutes Male — A B C: 7:00 7:45 8:30 Female — A B C: 9:00 9:45 10:45	Run 20 minutes Male — A B C: 7:00 7:45 8:30 Female — A B C: 9:00 9:45 10:45	Run 20 minutes Male — A B C: 7:00 7:30 8:15 Female — A B C: 9:00 9:30 10:30	Run 20 minutes Male — A B C: 7:00 7:30 8:15 Female — A B C: 9:00 9:30 10:30
	COOL-DOWN	SD	SD	SD	SD
TUESDAY	WARM-UP	4C, HSD & CD1	4C, HSD & CD1	4C, HSD & CD1	4C, HSD & CD1
	ACTIVITY	CD2 (10/10/5 reps x 2 sets) CD3 (5 reps x 1 set)	CD2 (10/10/5 reps x 2 sets) CD3 (5 reps x 1 set)	CD2 (15/15/5 reps x 1 set) CD3 (5 reps x 1 set)	CD2 (15/15/5 reps x 1 set) CD3 (5 reps x 1 set)
	COOL-DOWN	SD	SD	SD	SD
WEDNESDAY	WARM-UP	CD1 & MMD	CD1 & MMD	CD1 & MMD	CD1 & MMD
	ACTIVITY	30:60s (10 reps)	30:60s (10 reps)	30:60s (10 reps)	30:60s (10 reps)
	COOL-DOWN	SD	SD	SD	SD

TRAINING SCHEDULE 3
(continued)

		THURSDAY	FRIDAY	SATURDAY	
WEEK NINE	WARM-UP	4C, HSD & CD1	CD1 & MMD	REST	
	ACTIVITY	CD2 (10/10/5 reps x 2 sets)	Run 20 minutes		
		CD3 (5 reps x 1 set)	Male A B C		
			7:00 7:45 8:30		
			Female A B C		
			9:00 9:45 10:45		
	COOL-DOWN	SD	SD		
WEEK TEN	WARM-UP	4C, HSD & CD1	CD1 & MMD	REST	
	ACTIVITY	CD2 (10/10/5 reps x 2 sets)	Run 20 minutes		
		CD3 (5 reps x 1 set)	Male A B C		
			7:00 7:45 8:30		
			Female A B C		
			9:00 9:45 10:45		
	COOL-DOWN	SD	SD		
WEEK ELEVEN	WARM-UP	4C, HSD & CD1	CD1 & MMD	REST	
	ACTIVITY	CD2 (15/15/5 reps x 1 set)	Run 20 minutes		
		CD3 (5 reps x 1 set)	Male A B C		
			7:00 7:30 8:15		
			Female A B C		
			9:00 9:30 10:30		
	COOL-DOWN	SD	SD		
WEEK TWELVE	WARM-UP	4C, HSD & CD1			
	ACTIVITY	CD2 (15/15/5 reps x 1 set)	REST	1-1-1 PHYSICAL FITNESS ASSESSMENT	
		CD3 (5 reps x 1 set)			
	COOL-DOWN	SD			

YEAR

MONTH

TRAINING SCHEDULE 3
Maintenance Phase

	MONDAY	TUESDAY	WEDNESDAY	THURSDAY	FRIDAY
WARM-UP	CD1 & MMD	4C, HSD & CD1	CD1 & MMD	4C, HSD & CD1	CD1 & MMD
ACTIVITY	A & B Run 30 minutes	CD2 (15/15/5 reps x 2 sets)	30:60s (10 reps)	CD2 (15/15/5 reps x 2 sets)	A & B Run 30 minutes
	C Run 20 minutes	CD3 (5 reps x 1 set)		CD3 (5 reps x 1 set)	C Run 20 minutes
	A B C				A B C
	7:30 8:00 9:30				7:30 8:00 9:30
COOL-DOWN	SD	SD	SD	SD	SD

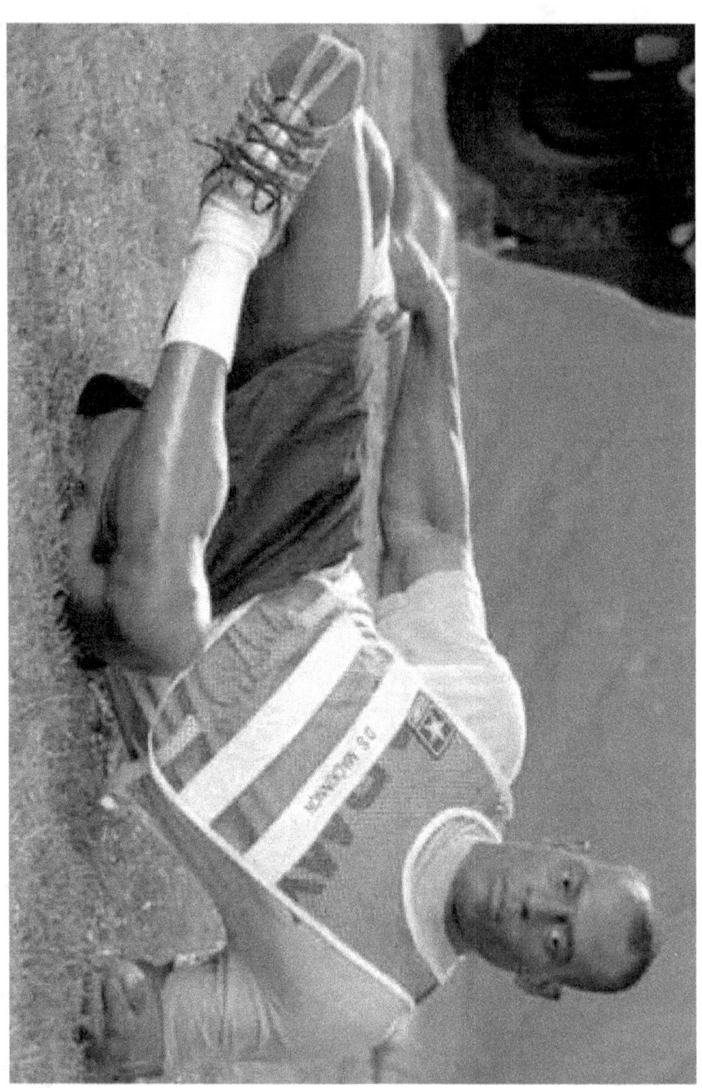

TRAINING SCHEDULE 4

		SUNDAY	MONDAY	TUESDAY	WEDNESDAY
WEEK ONE	WARM-UP	REST	CD1 & MMD	4C, HSD & CD1	CD1 & MMD
	ACTIVITY		Walk 4 min. Run 2 min. (5x)	CD2 (5/5/2 reps x 2 sets)	30:60s (4 reps)
	COOL-DOWN		SD	SD	SD
WEEK TWO	WARM-UP	REST	CD1 & MMD	4C, HSD & CD1	CD1 & MMD
	ACTIVITY		Walk 3 min. Run 3 min. (5x)	CD2 (6/6/3 reps x 2 sets)	30:60s (4 reps)
	COOL-DOWN		SD	SD	SD
WEEK THREE	WARM-UP	REST	CD1 & MMD	4C, HSD & CD1	CD1 & MMD
	ACTIVITY		Walk 2 min. Run 4 min. (5x)	CD2 7/7/4 reps x 2 sets)	30:60s (5 reps)
	COOL-DOWN		SD	SD	SD
WEEK FOUR	WARM-UP	REST	CD1 & MMD	4C, HSD & CD1	CD1 & MMD
	ACTIVITY		Walk 2 min. Run 4 min. (5x)	CD2 (8/8/4 reps x 2 sets)	30:60s (5 reps)
	COOL-DOWN		SD	SD	SD

TRAINING SCHEDULE 4
(continued)

Day	Week One			Week Two			Week Three			Week Four		
	WARM-UP	ACTIVITY	COOL-DOWN	WARM-UP	ACTIVITY	COOL-DOWN	WARM-UP	ACTIVITY	COOL-DOWN	WARM-UP	ACTIVITY	COOL-DOWN
THURSDAY	4C, HSD & CD1	CD2 (5/5/2 reps x 2 sets)	SD	4C, HSD & CD1	CD2 (6/6/3 reps x 2 sets)	SD	4C, HSD & CD1	CD2 7/7/4 reps x 2 sets)	SD	4C, HSD & CD1	CD2 (8/8/4 reps x 2 sets)	SD
FRIDAY	CD1 & MMD	Walk 4 min. Run 2 min. (5x)	SD	CD1 & MMD	Walk 3 min. Run 3 min. (5x)	SD	CD1 & MMD	Walk 2 min. Run 4 min. (5x)	SD	REST		
SATURDAY	REST			REST						1-1-1 PHYSICAL FITNESS ASSESSMENT		

MONTH　　　　**YEAR**

TRAINING SCHEDULE 4
(continued)

			SUNDAY	MONDAY	TUESDAY	WEDNESDAY
WEEK FIVE		WARM-UP	REST	CD1 & MMD	4C, HSD & CD1	CD1 & MMD
		ACTIVITY		Run 10 minutes	CD2 (10/10/5 reps x 1 set)	30:60s (6 reps)
					CD3 (5 reps x 1 set)	
		COOL-DOWN		SD	SD	SD
WEEK SIX		WARM-UP	REST	CD1 & MMD	4C, HSD & CD1	CD1 & MMD
		ACTIVITY		Run 12 minutes	CD2 (10/10/5 reps x 1 set)	30:60s (6 reps)
					CD3 (5 reps x 1 set)	
		COOL-DOWN		SD	SD	SD
WEEK SEVEN		WARM-UP	REST	CD1 & MMD	4C, HSD & CD1	CD1 & MMD
		ACTIVITY		Run 1 mile	CD2 (10/10/5 reps x 1 set)	30:60s (7 reps)
				M: 9:30/F: 11:30	CD3 (5 reps x 1 set)	
		COOL-DOWN		SD	SD	SD
WEEK EIGHT		WARM-UP	REST	CD1 & MMD	4C, HSD & CD1	CD1 & MMD
		ACTIVITY		Run 1 mile	CD2 (10/10/5 reps x 1 set)	30:60s (7 reps)
				M: 9:15/F: 11:15	CD3 (5 reps x 1 set)	
		COOL-DOWN		SD	SD	SD

TRAINING SCHEDULE 4
(continued)

		THURSDAY	FRIDAY	SATURDAY	
WEEK FIVE	WARM-UP	4C, HSD & CD1	CD1 & MMD	REST	YEAR
	ACTIVITY	CD2 (10/10/5 reps x 1 set)	Run 10 minutes		
		CD3 (5 reps x 1 set)			
	COOL-DOWN	SD	SD		
WEEK SIX	WARM-UP	4C, HSD & CD1	CD1 & MMD	REST	
	ACTIVITY	CD2 (10/10/5 reps x 1 set)	Run 12 minutes		
		CD3 (5 reps x 1 set)			
	COOL-DOWN	SD	SD		
WEEK SEVEN	WARM-UP	4C, HSD & CD1	CD1 & MMD	REST	MONTH
	ACTIVITY	CD2 (10/10/5 reps x 1 set)	Run 1 mile		
		CD3 (5 reps x 1 set)	M: 9:30/F: 11:30		
	COOL-DOWN	SD	SD		
WEEK EIGHT	WARM-UP	4C, HSD & CD1	REST	1-1-1 PHYSICAL FITNESS ASSESSMENT	
	ACTIVITY	CD2 (10/10/5 reps x 1 set)			
		CD3 (5 reps x 1 set)			
	COOL-DOWN	SD			

TRAINING SCHEDULE 4
(continued)

		SUNDAY	MONDAY	TUESDAY	WEDNESDAY
WEEK NINE	WARM-UP	REST	CD1 & MMD	4C, HSD & CD1	CD1 & MMD
	ACTIVITY		Run 1 mile	CD2 (10/10/5 reps x 2 sets)	30:60s (8 reps)
			M: 9:00/F: 11:00	CD3 (5 reps x 1 set)	
	COOL-DOWN		SD	SD	SD
WEEK TEN	WARM-UP	REST	CD1 & MMD	4C, HSD & CD1	CD1 & MMD
	ACTIVITY		Run 1 mile	CD2 (10/10/5 reps x 2 sets)	30:60s (8 reps)
			M: 8:45/F: 10:45	CD3 (5 reps x 1 set)	
	COOL-DOWN		SD	SD	SD
WEEK ELEVEN	WARM-UP	REST	CD1 & MMD	4C, HSD & CD1	CD1 & MMD
	ACTIVITY		Run 1 mile	CD2 (15/15/5 reps x 1 set)	30:60s (8 reps)
			M: 8:30/F: 10:30	CD3 (5 reps x 1 set)	
	COOL-DOWN		SD	SD	SD
WEEK TWELVE	WARM-UP	REST	CD1 & MMD	4C, HSD & CD1	CD1 & MMD
	ACTIVITY		Run 1 mile	CD2 (15/15/5 reps x 1 set)	30:60s (8 reps)
			M: 8:15/F: 10:15	CD3 (5 reps x 1 set)	
	COOL-DOWN		SD	SD	SD

			THURSDAY	FRIDAY	SATURDAY	
TRAINING SCHEDULE 4 (continued)	WEEK NINE	WARM-UP	4C, HSD & CD1	CD1 & MMD	REST	YEAR
		ACTIVITY	CD2 (10/10/5 reps x 2 sets)	Run 1 mile		
			CD3 (5 reps x 1 set)	M: 9:00/F: 11:00		
		COOL-DOWN	SD	SD		
	WEEK TEN	WARM-UP	4C, HSD & CD1	CD1 & MMD	REST	
		ACTIVITY	CD2 (10/10/5 reps x 2 sets)	Run 1 mile		
			CD3 (5 reps x 1 set)	M: 8:45/F: 10:45		
		COOL-DOWN	SD	SD		
	WEEK ELEVEN	WARM-UP	4C, HSD & CD1	CD1 & MMD	REST	MONTH
		ACTIVITY	CD2 (15/15/5 reps x 1 set)	Run 1 mile		
			CD3 (5 reps x 1 set)	M: 8:30/F: 10:30		
		COOL-DOWN	SD	SD		
	WEEK TWELVE	WARM-UP	4C, HSD & CD1	REST	1-1-1 PHYSICAL FITNESS ASSESSMENT	
		ACTIVITY	CD2 (15/15/5 reps x 1 set)			
			CD3 (5 reps x 1 set)			
		COOL-DOWN	SD			

TRAINING SCHEDULE 4
Maintenance Phase

	MONDAY	TUESDAY	WEDNESDAY	THURSDAY	FRIDAY
WARM-UP	CD1 & MMD	4C, HSD & CD1	CD1 & MMD	4C, HSD & CD1	CD1 & MMD
ACTIVITY	Run 20-30 minutes	CD2 (15/15/5 reps x 2 sets)	30:60s (10 reps)	CD2 (15/15/5 reps x 2 sets)	Run 20-30 minutes
		CD3 (5 reps x 1 set)		CD3 (5 reps x 1 set)	
COOL-DOWN	SD	SD	SD	SD	SD

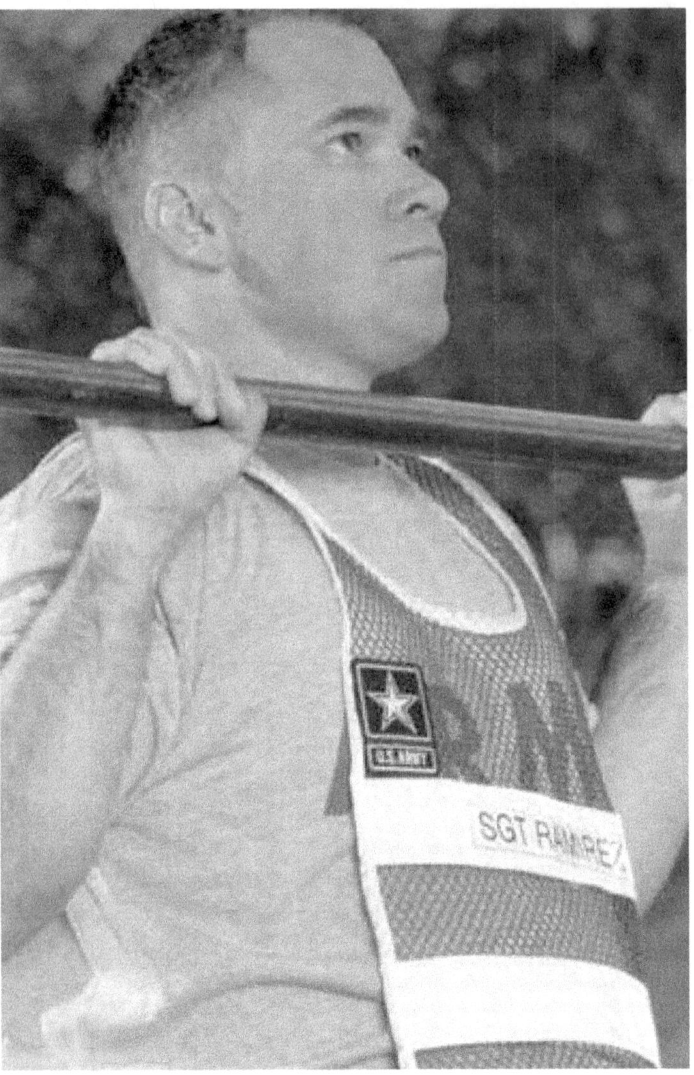

U.S. ARMY
SGT RAMIREZ

TRAINING SCHEDULE

	WEEK FOUR					WEEK THREE					WEEK TWO					WEEK ONE				
	WARM-UP	ACTIVITY			COOL-DOWN	WARM-UP	ACTIVITY			COOL-DOWN	WARM-UP	ACTIVITY			COOL-DOWN	WARM-UP	ACTIVITY			COOL-DOWN
SUNDAY																				
MONDAY																				
TUESDAY																				
WEDNESDAY																				

TRAINING SCHEDULE

	WEEK FOUR	WEEK THREE	WEEK TWO	WEEK ONE	
	WARM-UP / ACTIVITY / COOL-DOWN	WARM-UP / ACTIVITY / COOL-DOWN	WARM-UP / ACTIVITY / COOL-DOWN	WARM-UP / ACTIVITY / COOL-DOWN	THURSDAY
					FRIDAY
	REST				
	1-1-1 PHYSICAL FITNESS ASSESSMENT				SATURDAY

MONTH   YEAR

TRAINING SCHEDULE

	WEEK FIVE					WEEK SIX					WEEK SEVEN					WEEK EIGHT				
	WARM-UP	ACTIVITY			COOL-DOWN	WARM-UP	ACTIVITY			COOL-DOWN	WARM-UP	ACTIVITY			COOL-DOWN	WARM-UP	ACTIVITY			COOL-DOWN
SUNDAY																				
MONDAY																				
TUESDAY																				
WEDNESDAY																				

TRAINING SCHEDULE

WEEK EIGHT	WEEK SEVEN	WEEK SIX	WEEK FIVE	
WARM-UP / ACTIVITY / COOL-DOWN	WARM-UP / ACTIVITY / COOL-DOWN	WARM-UP / ACTIVITY / COOL-DOWN	WARM-UP / ACTIVITY / COOL-DOWN	
				THURSDAY
REST				FRIDAY
1-1-1 PHYSICAL FITNESS ASSESSMENT				SATURDAY

MONTH

YEAR

TRAINING SCHEDULE

WEEK TWELVE						WEEK ELEVEN						WEEK TEN						WEEK NINE					
WARM-UP	ACTIVITY				COOL-DOWN	WARM-UP	ACTIVITY				COOL-DOWN	WARM-UP	ACTIVITY				COOL-DOWN	WARM-UP	ACTIVITY				COOL-DOWN
																								SUNDAY
																								MONDAY
																								TUESDAY
																								WEDNESDAY

TRAINING SCHEDULE

	WEEK TWELVE				WEEK ELEVEN				WEEK TEN				WEEK NINE			
	WARM-UP	ACTIVITY			COOL-DOWN	WARM-UP	ACTIVITY			COOL-DOWN	WARM-UP	ACTIVITY			COOL-DOWN	WARM-UP	ACTIVITY			COOL-DOWN

THURSDAY

FRIDAY — REST

SATURDAY — 1-1-1 PHYSICAL FITNESS ASSESSMENT

MONTH | YEAR

PERSONAL TRAINING ASSESSMENTS

DATE	NUMBER OF PUSH-UPS	NUMBER OF SIT-UPS	1-MILE RUN TIME

PERSONAL TRAINING ASSESSMENTS

DATE	NUMBER OF PUSH-UPS	NUMBER OF SIT-UPS	1-MILE RUN TIME

★ WE STRIVE ★

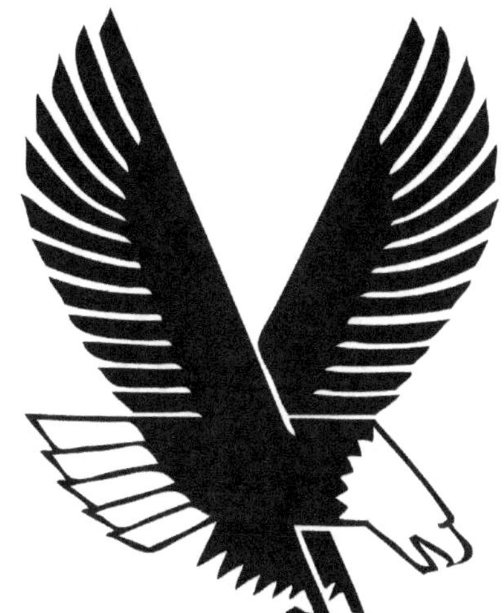

...To bring you
THE BEST
HOW-TO BOOKS
☆ IN THE WORLD ☆

**If you enjoyed this one,
please TAKE A MOMENT to
LEAVE A REVIEW at:**

★ **AMZN.COM/1979401985** ★